Table of Contents

Table of Contents ....

Introduction 15

Ketogenic Recipes for Breakfast 16

Poached Eggs 16
Breakfast Bowl 16
Eggs and Sausages 16
Scrambled Eggs 17
Frittata 17
Smoked Salmon Breakfast 17
Feta and Asparagus Delight 18
Eggs Baked in Avocados 18
Seasoned Hard-boiled Eggs 18
Shrimp and Bacon Breakfast 19
Mexican Breakfast 19
Breakfast Pie 19
Breakfast Stir-fry 20
Breakfast Skillet 20
Breakfast Casserole 20
Sausage Patties 21
Sausage Quiche 21
Baked Eggs with Sausage 21
Chorizo and Cauliflower Breakfast 22
Italian Spaghetti Casserole 22
Porridge 22
Granola 23
Almond Cereal 23
Nutty Breakfast Bowl 23
Breakfast Bread 24
Breakfast Muffins 24
Vegetable Breakfast Bread 24
Breadless Breakfast Sandwich 25
Chicken Breakfast Muffins 25
Herbed Biscuits 25
Avocado Muffins 26
Bacon and Lemon Thyme Muffins 26
Cheese and Oregano Muffins 26
Turkey Breakfast 27

Burrito 27

Breakfast Hash 27

Brussels Sprout Delight 28

Cereal Nibs 28

Chia Pudding 28

Hemp Porridge 29

Simple Breakfast Cereal 29

Simple Egg Porridge 29

Pancakes 30

Almond Pancakes 30

Pumpkin Pancakes 30

Simple French Toast 31

Waffles 31

Baked Granola 31

Nutty Breakfast Smoothie 32

Kiwi and Pineapple Smoothie 32

Breakfast in a Glass 32

Steak and Eggs 33

Chicken Quiche 33

Chicken Omelet 33

Simple Smoothie Bowl 34

Feta Omelet 34

Breakfast Meatloaf 34

Breakfast Tuna Salad 35

Breakfast Salad in a Jar 35

Naan Bread and Butter 35

Ketogenic Recipes for Lunch 36

Lunch Caesar Salad 36

Lunch Tacos 36

Lunch Pizza 36

Pizza Rolls 37

Cheese Dough Pizza 37

Taco Salad 38

Stuffed Peppers 38

Beef Brisket Burgers 38

Chili Pepper Burger 39

Zucchini with Cheese 39

Bacon and Zucchini Noodles Salad 39

Chicken Salad	40
Steak Salad	40
Fennel and Chicken Salad	40
Easy Stuffed Avocado	41
Pesto Chicken Salad	41
Chimichurri Steak Salad	41
Easy Crab Cakes	42
Lunch Muffins	42
Pork Pie	43
Lunch Pâte	43
Chicken Chowder	44
Coconut Soup	44
Zucchini Noodles Soup	45
Lunch Curry	45
Spinach Rolls	46
Steak Bowl	46
Meatball Pilaf	47
Broccoli Soup	47
Green Beans Salad	47
Pumpkin Soup	48
Green Bean Casserole	48
Apple Salad	49
Brussels Sprout Gratin	49
Fried Asparagus	49
Shrimp Pasta	50
Mexican Casserole	50
Asian Salad	50
Simple Buffalo Wings	51
Bacon and Mushrooms Skewers	51
Simple Tomato Soup	51
Bacon-wrapped Sausages	52
Lobster Bisque	52
Halloumi Salad	52
Beef Shank Stew	53
Chicken and Shrimp	53
Green Soup	54
Caprese Salad	54
Salmon Soup	54
Halibut Soup	55

Ketogenic Side Dish Recipes 56

Simple Kimchi 56
Oven-fried Green Beans 56
Cauliflower Mash 56
Portobello Mushrooms 57
Broiled Brussels Sprouts 57
Pesto 57
Brussels Sprouts and Bacon 58
Creamy Spinach 58
Avocado Fries 58
Roasted Cauliflower 59
Mushrooms and Spinach 59
Okra and Tomatoes 59
Snap Peas and Mint 60
Collard Greens with Turkey 60
Eggplant and Tomatoes 60
Broccoli with Lemon Almond Butter 61
Sautéed Broccoli 61
Easy Grilled Onions 61
Sautéed Zucchini 62
Fried Swiss Chard 62
Mushroom Salad 62
Greek Side Salad 63
Tomato Salsa 63
Summer Side Salad 63
Tomato and Bocconcini 64
Cucumber and Date Salad 64
Eggplant Salad 64
Baked Eggplant Side Salad 65
Endive and Watercress Side Salad 65
Indian Side Salad 65
Indian Mint Chutney 66
Indian Coconut Chutney 66
Easy Tamarind Chutney 66
Caramelized Bell Peppers 67
Caramelized Red Chard 67
Summer Kale 67
Coleslaw 68

Fried Cabbage 68

Green Beans and Avocado 68

Creamy Spaghetti Pasta 69

Roasted Olives 69

Vegetable Noodles 69

Mustard and Garlic Brussels Sprouts 70

Cheese Sauce 70

Sautéed Kohlrabi 70

Turnip Fries 71

Creamy Cauliflower and Spinach 71

Twice-baked Zucchini 71

Sausage Gravy 72

Mushroom and Hemp Pilaf 72

Asian Side Salad 72

Mixed Vegetable Dish 73

Cauliflower Polenta 73

Sausage Stuffing 74

Baby Mushrooms 74

Green Beans with Vinaigrette 75

Braised Asian Eggplant 75

Cheddar Soufflés 75

Cauliflower Side Salad 76

Rice with Cauliflower 76

Ketogenic Snacks and Appetizers Recipes 77

Marinated Eggs 77

Sausage and Cheese Dip 77

Onion and Cauliflower Dip 77

Pesto Crackers 78

Pumpkin Muffins 78

Special Tortilla Chips 78

Jalapeño Balls 79

Pepperoni Bombs 79

Cheeseburger Muffins 79

Pizza Dip 80

Flaxseed and Almond Muffins 80

Fried Queso 80

Maple and Pecan Bars 81

Baked Chia Seeds 81

Simple Tomato Tarts 82
Avocado Dip 82
Prosciutto-wrapped Shrimp 82
Broccoli and Cheddar Biscuits 83
Corndogs 83
Mini Bell Pepper Nachos 83
Almond Butter Bars 84
Saucy Zucchini 84
Zucchini Chips 84
Simple Hummus 85
Celery Sticks 85
Beef Jerky 85
Crab Dip 86
Spinach Balls 86
Garlic Spinach Dip 86
Stuffed Mushrooms 87
Breadsticks 87
Italian Meatballs 87
Parmesan Wings 88
Cheese Sticks 88
Broccoli Sticks 88
Bacon Delight 89
Taco Cups 89
Chicken Egg Rolls 89
Cheese Fries 90
Jalapeño Crisps 90
Cucumber Cups 90
Caviar Salad 91
Marinated Kebabs 91
Zucchini Rolls 91
Green Crackers 92
Cheese and Pesto Terrine 92
Avocado Salsa 92
Egg Chips 93
Chili Lime Chips 93
Artichoke Dip 93

Ketogenic Fish and Seafood Recipes 94

Fish Pie 94

Baked Haddock 94
Tilapia 95
Trout with Special Sauce 95
Trout with Butter Sauce 95
Roasted Salmon 96
Salmon Meatballs 96
Salmon with Caper Sauce 96
Simple Grilled Oysters 97
Baked Halibut 97
Crusted Salmon 97
Sour Cream Salmon 98
Grilled Salmon 98
Tuna Cakes 98
Pan-roasted Cod 99
Sea Bass with Capers 99
Cod with Arugula 99
Baked Halibut with Vegetables 100
Fish Curry 100
Sautéed Lemon Shrimp 100
Roasted Sea Bass 101
Coconut Shrimp 101
Shrimp and Noodle Salad 101
Roasted Mahi Mahi and Salsa 102
Spicy Shrimp 102
Shrimp Stew 102
Shrimp Alfredo 103
Shrimp and Snow Pea Soup 103
Garlicky Mussels 103
Fried Calamari with Spicy Sauce 104
Baked Calamari and Shrimp 104
Octopus Salad 104
Clam Chowder 105
Flounder and Shrimp 105
Shrimp Salad 106
Fiery Oysters 106
Salmon Rolls 106
Salmon Skewers 107
Grilled Shrimp 107
Calamari Salad 107

Cod Salad 108

Sardine Salad 108

Italian Clams Delight 108

Orange-glazed Salmon 109

Tuna and Chimichurri Sauce 109

Salmon Bites with Chili Sauce 110

Irish Clams 110

Seared Scallops with Walnuts and Grapes 111

Oysters with Pico De Gallo 111

Grilled Squid with Guacamole 112

Shrimp and Cauliflower 112

Salmon Stuffed with Shrimp 113

Mustard-glazed Salmon 113

Salmon with Arugula and Cabbage 113

Scallops with Fennel Sauce 114

Salmon with Lemon Relish 114

Mussel Soup 114

Swordfish with Mango Salsa 115

Sushi Bowl 115

Grilled Swordfish 116

Ketogenic Poultry Recipes 117

Chicken Nuggets 117

Chicken Wings with Mint Chutney 117

Chicken Meatballs 118

Grilled Chicken Wings 118

Easy Baked Chicken 118

Italian Chicken 119

Lemon Chicken 119

Fried Chicken with Paprika Sauce 119

Chicken Fajitas 120

Skillet Chicken and Mushrooms 120

Chicken with Olive Tapenade 121

Pan-seared Duck Breast 121

Duck Breast with Vegetables 121

Duck Breast Salad 122

Turkey Pie 122

Turkey Soup 123

Baked Turkey Delight 123

Turkey Chili 123
Turkey and Tomato Curry 124
Turkey and Cranberry Salad 124
Stuffed Chicken Breast 124
Chicken with Mustard Sauce 125
Salsa Chicken 125
Italian Chicken 125
Chicken Casserole 126
Chicken-stuffed Peppers 126
Creamy Chicken 126
Chicken and Broccoli Casserole 127
Creamy Chicken Soup 127
Chicken Crepes 128
Four-cheese Chicken 128
Crusted Chicken 129
Cheesy Chicken 129
Orange Chicken 130
Chicken Pie 130
Bacon-wrapped Chicken 131
Red-hot Chicken Wings 131
Chicken in Creamy Sauce 131
Savory Chicken 132
Chicken with Sour Cream Sauce 132
Chicken Stroganoff 132
Chicken Gumbo 133
Chicken Thighs with Mushrooms and Cheese 133
Pecan-crusted Chicken 133
Pepperoni Chicken Bake 134
Fried Chicken 134
Chicken Calzone 134
Mexican Chicken Soup 135
Simple Chicken Stir-fry 135
Spinach and Artichoke Chicken 135
Chicken Meatloaf 136
One-pot Roasted Chicken 136
Chicken with Green Onion Sauce 136
Chicken-stuffed Mushrooms 137
Chicken-stuffed Avocados 137
Balsamic Chicken 137

Chicken Pasta 138
Peanut-grilled Chicken 138
Chicken Stew 139
Chicken and Vegetable Stew 139

Ketogenic Meat Recipes 140

Roasted Pork Belly 140
Stuffed Pork 140
Pork Chops with Mushrooms 141
Italian Pork Rolls 141
Lemon and Garlic Pork 142
Jamaican Pork 142
Cranberry Pork Roast 142
Juicy Pork Chops 142
Lemon Pork Chops 143
Mediterranean Pork 143
Italian Pork Chops 144
Spicy Pork Chops 144
Thai Beef 144
Beef Patties 145
Beef Pot Roast 145
Beef Zucchini Cups 145
Beef Meatball Casserole 146
Beef and Tomato-stuffed Squash 146
Beef Chili 147
Glazed Beef Meatloaf 147
Beef with Tzatziki 148
Meatballs with Mushroom Sauce 148
Beef and Sauerkraut Soup 149
Ground Beef Casserole 149
Zucchini Noodles and Beef 150
Jamaican Beef Pies 150
Beef Goulash 151
Beef and Eggplant Casserole 151
Braised Lamb Chops 152
Lamb Salad 152
Moroccan Lamb 153
Lamb with Mustard Sauce 153
Lamb Curry 154

Lamb Stew 154
Lamb Casserole 155
Slow-cooked Leg of Lamb 155
Lavender Lamb Chops 155
Paprika Lamb Chops 156
Lamb with Orange Dressing 156
Lamb Riblets and Mint Pesto 156
Lamb with Fennel and Figs 157
Baked Veal and Cabbage 157
Beef Bourguignon 157
Slow-roasted Beef 158
Beef Stew 158
Pork Stew 158
Sausage Stew 159
Burgundy Beef Stew 159
Cuban Beef Stew 160
Ham Stew 160
Veal Stew 160
Veal with Tomatoes 161
Veal Parmesan 161
Veal Piccata 161
Roasted Pork Sausage 162
Baked Sausage and Kale 162
Sausage with Tomatoes and Cheese 162
Sausage Salad 163
Sausage and Peppers Soup 163
Italian Sausage Soup 163

Ketogenic Vegetable Recipes 164

Puréed Broccoli and Cauliflower 164
Broccoli Stew 164
Watercress Soup 164
Bok Choy Soup 165
Bok Choy Stir-fry 165
Cream of Celery Soup 165
Celery Soup 166
Celery Stew 166
Spinach Soup 166
Sautéed Mustard Greens 167

Collard Greens and Ham 167
Collard Greens and Tomatoes 167
Sautéed Mustard Greens 168
Collard Greens and Poached Eggs 168
Collard Greens Soup 168
Spring Greens Soup 169
Mustard Greens and Spinach Soup 169
Roasted Asparagus 169
Asparagus Fries 170
Asparagus and Browned Butter 170
Asparagus Frittata 170
Creamy Asparagus 171
Alfalfa Sprouts Salad 171
Roasted Radishes 171
Radish Hash Browns 172
Crispy Radishes 172
Creamy Radishes 172
Radish Soup 173
Avocado Salad 173
Avocado and Egg Salad 173
Avocado and Cucumber Salad 174
Avocado Soup 174
Avocado and Bacon Soup 174
Thai Avocado Soup 175
Arugula Salad 175
Arugula Soup 175
Arugula and Broccoli Soup 176
Zucchini Cream 176
Zucchini and Avocado Soup 176
Swiss Chard Pie 177
Swiss Chard Salad 177
Green Salad 177
Catalan-style Greens 178
Swiss Chard and Chicken Soup 178
Swiss Chard and Vegetable Soup 179
Roasted Tomato Cream 179
Eggplant Soup 180
Eggplant Stew 180
Roasted Bell Peppers Soup 180

 Cabbage Soup 181
Ketogenic Dessert Recipes 182
 Chocolate Truffles 182
 Doughnuts 182
 Chocolate Bombs 182
 Gelatin 183
 Strawberry Pie 183
 Chocolate Pie 184
 Mini Cheesecakes 184
 Raspberry and Coconut Dessert 185
 Chocolate Cups 185
 Berry Mousse 185
 Peanut Butter Fudge 186
 Lemon Mousse 186
 Vanilla Ice Cream 186
 Cheesecake Squares 187
 Brownies 187
 Chocolate Pudding 187
 Vanilla Parfaits 188
 Avocado Pudding 188
 Mint Delight 188
 Coconut Pudding 189
 Creamy Coconut Pudding 189
 Chocolate Biscotti 189
 Peanut Butter and Chocolate Brownies 190
 Blueberry Scones 190
 Chocolate Cookies 190
 Orange Cake 191
 Walnut Spread 191
 Mug Cake 191
 Sweet Buns 192
 Lemon Custard 192
 Chocolate Ganache 192
 Mixed Berries and Cream 193
 Coconut Ice Cream 193
 Macaroons 193
 Lime Cheesecake 194
 Coconut and Strawberries 194

- *Caramel Custard* **194**
- *Cookie Dough Balls* **195**
- *Ricotta Mousse* **195**
- *Coconut Granola* **195**
- *Peanut Butter and Chia Pudding* **196**
- *Pumpkin Custard* **196**
- *No-bake Cookies* **196**
- *Butter Delight* **197**
- *Marshmallows* **197**
- *Tiramisu Pudding* **197**
- *Summer Smoothie* **198**
- *Lemon Sorbet* **198**
- *Raspberry Ice Pops* **198**
- *Cherry and Chia Jam* **198**

Conclusion **199**

Introduction

Do you want to make a change in your life? Do you want to become a healthier person who can enjoy a new and improved life? If so, you are definitely in the right place. You are about to discover a wonderful and healthy diet that has changed millions of lives. The diet we are talking about the ketogenic diet, which is more of a lifestyle than a diet, one that will mesmerize you and make you feel a new person in no time. Here is everything you need to know and about the ketogenic diet.

A keto diet is a low-carb diet. During such a diet, your body makes ketones in your liver, and these are used as energy. As a result, your body produces less insulin and glucose and a state of ketosis is induced.

Ketosis is a natural process that appears when food intake is lower than usual. The body will soon adapt to this state and, therefore, you will be able to lose weight in no time. In addition, you will also become healthier and your physical and mental performances will improve.

Your blood sugar levels will improve, and you won't be predisposed to diabetes. Additionally, epilepsy and heart disease can be prevented if you are on a ketogenic diet.
Your cholesterol will improve, and you will feel amazing in no time.

A ketogenic diet is simple and to follow as long as you follow some simple rules. You don't need to make huge changes but there are some things you should know.

If you are on a ketogenic diet, there are certain foods that you must avoid at all times:
- Grains like corn, cereals, and rice
- Fruits like bananas, oranges, and grapes
- Sugar
- Dried beans
- Honey, and similar sweeteners
- Potatoes, and yams

However, if you are on a ketogenic diet you can eat:
- Greens like spinach, green beans, and kale
- Meat like poultry, fish, and pork
- Eggs
- Vegetables that grow above-ground vegetables like cauliflower, broccoli, and napa cabbage
- Nuts and seeds
- Cheese
- Butter
- Avocados
- Berries like strawberries, raspberries, and blueberries
- Sugar substitutes like erythritol, sucralose, and stevia
- Cooking oils like coconut oil, avocado oil, and olive oil

The list of foods you are allowed to eat on a keto diet is permissive and rich as you can see for yourself. Therefore, it should be easy for you to start such a diet.

If you've made this choice already, then it's time you checked our amazing keto recipe collection. You will discover 500 of the best ketogenic recipes around, and you will soon be able to make every one of these recipes - and even experiment with variations of your own.

Now, let's start your new magical culinary journey. Ketogenic lifestyle - here we come.

Ketogenic Recipes for Breakfast

Poached Eggs

Preparation time: 10 minutes
Cooking time: 35 minutes
Servings: 4

Ingredients:
- 3 garlic cloves, peeled and minced
- 1 tablespoon butter
- 1 white onion, peeled and chopped
- 1 Serrano pepper, chopped
- Salt and ground black pepper, to taste
- 1 red bell pepper, seeded and chopped
- 3 tomatoes, cored and chopped
- 1 teaspoon paprika
- 1 teaspoon cumin
- ¼ teaspoon chili powder
- 1 tablespoon fresh cilantro, chopped
- 6 eggs

Directions:
Heat up a pan with the butter over medium heat, add the onion, stir, and cook for 10 minutes. Add the Serrano pepper and garlic, stir, and cook for 1 minute. Add the red bell pepper, stir, and cook for 10 minutes. Add the tomatoes, salt, pepper, chili powder, cumin, and paprika, stir, and cook for 10 minutes. Crack the eggs into the pan, season them with salt, and pepper, cover pan, and cook for 6 minutes. Sprinkle cilantro at the end and serve.

Nutrition: Calories - 300, Fat - 12, Fiber - 3. 4, Carbs - 22, Protein - 14

Breakfast Bowl

Preparation time: 10 minutes
Cooking time: 20 minutes
Servings: 1

Ingredients:
- 4 ounces ground beef
- 1 onion, peeled and chopped
- 8 mushrooms, sliced
- Salt and ground black pepper, to taste
- 2 eggs, whisked
- 1 tablespoon coconut oil
- ½ teaspoon smoked paprika
- 1 avocado, pitted, peeled, and chopped
- 12 black olives, pitted and sliced

Directions:
Heat up a pan with the coconut oil over medium heat, add the onions, mushrooms, salt, and pepper, stir, and cook for 5 minutes. Add the beef, and paprika, stir, cook for 10 minutes, and transfer to a bowl. Heat up the pan again over medium heat, add the eggs, some salt, and pepper, and scramble them. Return beef mixture to pan and stir. Add the avocado and olives, stir, and cook for 1 minute. Transfer to a bowl and serve.

Nutrition: Calories - 600, Fat - 23, Fiber - 8, Carbs - 22, Protein - 43

Eggs and Sausages

Preparation time: 10 minutes
Cooking time: 35 minutes
Servings: 6

Ingredients:
- 5 tablespoons butter
- 12 eggs
- Salt and ground black pepper, to taste
- 1 ounce spinach, torn
- 12 ham slices
- 2 sausages, chopped
- 1 onion, peeled and chopped
- 1 red bell pepper, seeded and chopped

Directions:
Heat up a pan with 1 tablespoon butter over medium heat, add the sausages and onion, stir, and cook for 5 minutes. Add the bell pepper, salt, and pepper, stir, and cook for 3 minutes, and transfer to a bowl. Melt the rest of the butter, and divide into 12 cupcake molds. Add a slice of ham to each cupcake mold, divide the spinach in each and then the sausage mixture. Crack an egg on top, place in an oven, and bake at 425 degrees Fahrenheit for 20 minutes. Let them cool briefly before serving.

Nutrition: Calories - 440, Fat - 32, Fiber - 0, Carbs - 12, Protein - 22

Scrambled Eggs

Preparation time: 10 minutes
Cooking time: 10 minutes
Servings: 1

Ingredients:
- 4 bell mushrooms, chopped
- 3 eggs, whisked
- Salt and ground black pepper, to taste
- 2 ham slices, chopped
- ¼ cup red bell pepper, seeded and chopped
- ½ cup spinach, chopped
- 1 tablespoon coconut oil

Directions:
Heat up a pan with half of the oil over medium heat, add the mushrooms, spinach, ham, and bell pepper, stir, and cook for 4 minutes. Heat up another pan with the rest of the oil over medium heat, add the eggs, and scramble them. Add the vegetables, ham, salt, and pepper, stir, cook for 1 minute, and serve.

Nutrition: Calories - 350, Fat - 23, Fiber - 1, Carbs - 5, Protein - 22

Frittata

Preparation time: 10 minutes
Cooking time: 1 hour
Servings: 4

Ingredients:
- 9 ounces spinach
- 12 eggs
- 1 ounce pepperoni
- 1 teaspoon garlic, minced
- Salt and ground black pepper, to taste
- 5 ounces mozzarella cheese, shredded
- ½ cup Parmesan cheese, grated
- ½ cup ricotta cheese
- 4 tablespoons olive oil
- A pinch of nutmeg

Directions:
Squeeze liquid from spinach and put the spinach in a bowl. In another bowl, mix the eggs with salt, pepper, nutmeg, and garlic, and whisk. Add the spinach, Parmesan cheese, and ricotta cheese, and whisk. Pour this mixture into a pan, sprinkle with mozzarella cheese and pepperoni on top, place in an oven, and bake at 375°F for 45 minutes. Let the Let the frittata cool down for a few minutes before serving.

Nutrition: Calories - 298, Fat - 2, Fiber - 1, Carbs - 6, Protein - 18

Smoked Salmon Breakfast

Preparation time: 10 minutes
Cooking time: 10 minutes
Servings: 3

Ingredients:
- 4 eggs, whisked
- ½ teaspoon avocado oil
- 4 ounces smoked salmon, chopped
  For the sauce:
- 1 cup coconut milk
- ½ cup cashews, soaked and drained
- ¼ cup green onions, chopped
- 1 teaspoon garlic powder
- Salt and ground black pepper, to taste
- 1 tablespoon lemon juice

Directions:
In a blender, mix the cashews with coconut milk, garlic powder, and lemon juice and blend well. Add the salt, pepper, and green onions, blend again, transfer to a bowl, and place it in the refrigerator. Heat up a pan with the oil over medium-low heat, add the eggs, whisk, and cook until they are almost done. Place under a preheated broiler, and cook until the eggs are set. Divide the eggs on plates, top with smoked salmon, and serve with the green onion sauce on top.

Nutrition: Calories - 200, Fat - 10, Fiber - 2, Carbs - 11, Protein - 15

Feta and Asparagus Delight

Preparation time: 10 minutes
Cooking time: 25 minutes
Servings: 2

Ingredients:
- 12 asparagus spears
- 1 tablespoon olive oil
- 2 green onions, chopped
- 1 garlic clove, peeled and minced
- 6 eggs
- Salt and ground black pepper, to taste
- ½ cup feta cheese

Directions:
Heat up a pan with some water over medium heat, add the asparagus, cook for 8 minutes, drain well, chop 2 spears, and reserve the rest. Heat up a pan with the oil over medium heat, add the garlic, chopped asparagus, and onions, stir, and cook for 5 minutes. Add the eggs, salt, and pepper, stir, cover, and cook for 5 minutes. Arrange the asparagus spears on top of the frittata, sprinkle cheese, place in an oven at 350°F, and bake for 9 minutes. Divide on plates and serve.

Nutrition: Calories - 340, Fat - 12, Fiber - 3, Carbs - 8, Protein - 26

Eggs Baked in Avocados

Preparation time: 10 minutes
Cooking time: 20 minutes
Servings: 4

Ingredients:
- 2 avocados, cut in half and pitted
- 4 eggs
- Salt and ground black pepper, to taste
- 1 tablespoon fresh chives, chopped

Directions:
Scoop some flesh from the avocado halves, and arrange them in a baking dish. Crack an egg in each avocado, season with salt, and pepper, introduce them in the oven at 425°F, and bake for 20 minutes. Sprinkle chives at the end and serve.

Nutrition: Calories - 400, Fat - 34, Fiber - 13, Carbs - 13, Protein - 15

Seasoned Hard-boiled Eggs

Preparation time: 10 minutes
Cooking time: 4 minutes
Servings: 12

Ingredients:
- 4 tea bags
- 4 tablespoons salt
- 12 eggs
- 2 tablespoons ground cinnamon
- 6 star anise
- 1 teaspoon ground black pepper
- 1 tablespoons peppercorns
- 8 cups water
- 1 cup tamari sauce

Directions:
Put water in a pot, add the eggs, bring them to a boil over medium heat, and cook until they are hard boiled.
Cool them down, and crack them without peeling. In a large pot, mix water with tea bags, salt, pepper, peppercorns, cinnamon, star anise, and tamari sauce. Add the cracked eggs, cover pot, bring to a simmer over low heat, and cook for 30 minutes. Discard tea bags, and cook eggs for 3 hours and 30 minutes. Let the eggs to cool down, peel, and serve them.

Nutrition: Calories - 90, Fat - 6, Fiber - 0, Carbs - 0, Protein - 7

Shrimp and Bacon Breakfast

Preparation time: 10 minutes
Cooking time: 15 minutes
Servings: 4

Ingredients:
- 1 cup mushrooms, sliced
- 4 bacon slices, chopped
- 4 ounces smoked salmon, chopped
- 4 ounces shrimp, deveined
- Salt and ground black pepper, to taste
- ½ cup coconut cream

Directions:
Heat up a pan over medium heat, add the bacon, stir, and cook for 5 minutes. Add the mushrooms, stir, and cook for 5 minutes. Add the salmon, stir, and cook for 3 minutes. Add the shrimp, and cook for 2 minutes. Add the salt, pepper, and coconut cream, stir, cook for 1 minute, take off the heat, and divide on plates.

Nutrition: Calories - 340, Fat - 23, Fiber - 1, Carbs - 4, Protein - 17

Mexican Breakfast

Preparation time: 10 minutes
Cooking time: 30 minutes
Servings: 8

Ingredients:
- ½ cup enchilada sauce
- 1 pound ground pork
- 1 pound chorizo, chopped
- Salt and ground black pepper, to taste
- 8 eggs
- 1 tomato, cored and chopped
- 3 tablespoons butter
- ½ cup onion, chopped
- 1 avocado, pitted, peeled, and chopped

Directions:
In a bowl, mix the pork with chorizo, stir, and spread on a lined baking sheet. Spread enchilada sauce on top, place in an oven at 350ºF, and bake for 20 minutes. Heat up a pan with the butter over medium heat, add the eggs, and scramble them. Take the pork mixture out of the oven and spread the scrambled eggs over them. Sprinkle the salt, pepper, tomato, onion, and avocado on top, divide on plates, and serve.

Nutrition: Calories - 400, Fat - 32, Fiber - 4, Carbs - 7, Protein - 25

Breakfast Pie

Preparation time: 10 minutes
Cooking time: 45 minutes
Servings: 8

Ingredients:
- ½ onion, peeled and chopped
- 1 pie crust
- ½ red bell pepper, seeded and chopped
- ¾ pound ground beef
- Salt and ground black pepper, to taste
- 3 tablespoons taco seasoning
- ½ cup fresh cilantro, chopped
- 8 eggs
- 1 teaspoon coconut oil
- 1 teaspoon baking soda
- Mango salsa, for serving

Directions:
Heat up a pan with the oil over medium heat, add the beef, cook until it browns, and mix with salt, pepper, and taco seasoning. Stir again, transfer to a bowl, and set aside. Heat up the pan again over medium heat with cooking juices from the meat, add the onion and bell pepper, stir, and cook for 4 minutes. Add the eggs, baking soda, and some salt, and stir well. Add the cilantro, stir again, and take off the heat. Spread the beef mixture in pie crust, add the vegetables mixture, and spread over meat, place in an oven at 350ºF, and bake for 45 minutes. Let the pie cool, slice, divide on plates, and serve with mango salsa on top.

Nutrition: Calories - 198, Fat - 11, Fiber - 1, Carbs - 12, Protein - 12

Breakfast Stir-fry

Preparation time: 10 minutes
Cooking time: 30 minutes
Servings: 2

Ingredients:
- ½ pounds minced beef
- 2 teaspoons red chili flakes
- 1 tablespoon tamari sauce
- 2 bell peppers, seeded and chopped
- 1 teaspoon chili powder
- 1 tablespoon coconut oil
- Salt and ground black pepper, to taste

For the bok choy:
- 6 bunches bok choy, trimmed and chopped
- 1 teaspoon fresh ginger, grated
- Salt, to taste
- 1 tablespoon coconut oil

For the eggs:
- 1 tablespoon coconut oil
- 2 eggs

Directions:
Heat up a pan with 1 tablespoon coconut oil over medium-high heat, add the beef and bell peppers, stir, and cook for 10 minutes. Add the salt, pepper, tamari sauce, chili flakes, and chili powder, stir, cook for 4 minutes, and take off the heat. Heat up another pan with 1 tablespoon oil over medium heat, add the bok choy, stir, and cook for 3 minutes. Add the salt, and ginger, stir, cook for 2 minutes, and take off the heat. Heat up the third pan with 1 tablespoon oil over medium heat, crack the eggs, and fry them. Divide the beef and bell pepper mixture into 2 bowls. Divide the bok choy and top with the eggs.

Nutrition: Calories - 248, Fat - 14, Fiber - 4, Carbs - 10, Protein - 14

Breakfast Skillet

Preparation time: 10 minutes
Cooking time: 30 minutes
Servings: 4

Ingredients:
- 8 ounces mushrooms, chopped
- Salt and ground black pepper, to taste
- 1 pound minced pork
- 1 tablespoon coconut oil
- ½ teaspoon garlic powder
- ½ teaspoon dried basil
- 2 tablespoons Dijon mustard
- 2 zucchini, chopped

Directions:
Heat up a pan with the oil over medium-high heat, add the mushrooms, stir, and cook for 4 minutes. Add the zucchini, salt, and pepper, stir, and cook for 4 minutes. Add the pork, garlic powder, basil, and more salt and pepper, stir, and cook until meat is done. Add the mustard, stir, cook for 3 minutes, divide into bowls, and serve.

Nutrition: Calories - 240, Fat - 15, Fiber - 2, Carbs - 9, Protein - 17

Breakfast Casserole

Preparation time: 10 minutes
Cooking time: 40 minutes
Servings: 4

Ingredients:
- 10 eggs
- 1 pound pork sausage, chopped
- 1 onion, peeled and chopped
- 3 cups spinach, torn
- Salt and ground black pepper, to taste
- 3 tablespoons avocado oil

Directions:
Heat up a pan with 1 tablespoon oil over medium heat, add the sausage, stir, and brown it for 4 minutes.
Add the onion, stir, and cook for 3 minutes. Add the spinach, stir, and cook for 1 minute. Grease a baking dish with the rest of the oil, and spread the sausage mixture in it. Whisk the eggs, and add them to sausage mixture. Stir gently, place in an oven at 350°F, and bake for 30 minutes. Let the casserole cool for a few minutes before serving.

Nutrition: Calories - 345, Fat - 12, Fiber - 1, Carbs - 8, Protein - 22

Sausage Patties

Preparation time: 10 minutes
Cooking time: 10 minutes
Servings: 4

Ingredients:
- 1 pound minced pork
- Salt and ground black pepper, to taste
- ¼ teaspoon dried thyme
- ½ teaspoon dried sage
- ¼ teaspoon ground ginger
- 3 tablespoon cold water
- 1 tablespoon coconut oil

Directions:
Put the meat in a bowl. In another bowl, mix the water with salt, pepper, sage, thyme, and ginger, and whisk. Add this to the meat, and stir well. Shape the patties and place them on a working surface. Heat up a pan with the coconut oil over medium-high heat, add the patties, fry them for 5 minutes, flip, and cook them for 3 minutes. Serve warm.

Nutrition: Calories - 320, Fat - 13, Fiber - 2, Carbs - 10, Protein - 12

Sausage Quiche

Preparation time: 10 minutes
Cooking time: 40 minutes
Servings: 6

Ingredients:
- 12 ounces pork sausage, chopped
- Salt and ground black pepper, to taste
- 2 teaspoons whipping cream
- 2 tablespoons fresh parsley, chopped
- 10 mixed cherry tomatoes, halved
- 6 eggs
- 2 tablespoons Parmesan cheese, grated
- 5 eggplant slices

Directions:
Spread the sausage pieces on the bottom of a baking dish. Lay the eggplant slices on top and add the cherry tomatoes. In a bowl, mix the eggs with salt, pepper, cream, and Parmesan cheese, and whisk. Pour this into the baking dish, place in an oven at 375°F, bake for 40 minutes, and serve.

Nutrition: Calories - 340, Fat - 28, Fiber - 3, Carbs - 3, Protein - 17

Baked Eggs with Sausage

Preparation time: 10 minutes
Cooking time: 40 minutes
Servings: 6

Ingredients:
- 1 pound sausage, chopped
- 1 leek, chopped
- 8 eggs, whisked
- ¼ cup coconut milk
- 6 asparagus stalks, chopped
- 1 tablespoon fresh dill, chopped
- Salt and ground black pepper, to taste
- ¼ teaspoon garlic powder
- 1 tablespoon coconut oil, melted

Directions:
Heat up a pan over medium heat, add the sausage pieces, and brown them for a few minutes. Add the asparagus and leek, stir, and cook for a few minutes. In a bowl, mix the eggs with the salt, pepper, dill, garlic powder, and coconut milk, and whisk. Pour this into a baking dish greased with coconut oil. Add the sausage and vegetables on top and whisk them. Place in an oven at 325°F and bake for 40 minutes. Serve warm.

Nutrition: Calories - 340, Fat - 12, Fiber - 3, Carbs - 8, Protein - 23

Chorizo and Cauliflower Breakfast

Preparation time: 10 minutes
Cooking time: 45 minutes
Servings: 4

Ingredients:
- 1 pound chorizo, chopped
- 12 ounces canned green chilies, chopped
- 1 onion, peeled and chopped
- ½ teaspoon garlic powder
- Salt and ground black pepper, to taste
- 1 cauliflower head, separated into florets
- 4 eggs, whisked
- 2 tablespoons green onions, chopped

Directions:
Heat up a pan over medium heat, add the chorizo, and onion, stir, and brown for a few minutes. Add the green chilies, stir, cook for a few minutes, and take off the heat. In a food processor, mix the cauliflower with some salt and pepper and blend. Transfer this to a bowl, add the eggs, salt, pepper, garlic powder, and chorizo mixture, whisk, and transfer to a greased baking dish. Bake in the oven at 375°F for 40 minutes. Let the casserole cool down for a few minutes, sprinkle green onions on top, slice, and serve.

Nutrition: Calories - 350, Fat - 12, Fiber - 4, Carbs - 6, Protein - 20

Italian Spaghetti Casserole

Preparation time: 10 minutes
Cooking time: 55 minutes
Servings: 4

Ingredients:
- 4 tablespoons butter
- 1 spaghetti squash, halved
- Salt and ground black pepper, to taste
- ½ cup tomatoes, cored and chopped
- 2 garlic cloves, peeled and minced
- 1 cup onion, peeled and chopped
- ½ teaspoon Italian seasoning
- 3 ounces Italian salami, chopped
- ½ cup Kalamata olives, chopped
- 4 eggs
- ½ cup fresh parsley, chopped

Directions:
Place the squash halves on a lined baking sheet, season with salt and pepper, spread 1 tablespoon butter over them, place in an oven at 400°F, and bake for 45 minutes. Heat up a pan with the rest of the butter over medium heat, add the garlic, onions, salt, and pepper, stir, and cook for a couple of minutes. Add the salami and tomatoes, stir, and cook for 10 minutes. Add the olives, stir, and cook for a few minutes. Take the squash halves out of the oven, scrape the flesh with a fork, and add with the salami mixture to the pan. Stir, make 4 spaces in the mixture, crack an egg in each, season with salt, and pepper, place pan in the oven at 400°F, and bake until eggs are done. Sprinkle parsley on top and serve.

Nutrition: Calories - 333, Fat - 23, Fiber - 4, Carbs - 12, Protein - 15

Porridge

Preparation time: 5 minutes
Cooking time: 10 minutes
Servings: 1

Ingredients:
- 1 teaspoon ground cinnamon
- A pinch of nutmeg
- ½ cup almonds, ground
- 1 teaspoon stevia
- ¾ cup coconut cream
- A pinch of ground cardamom
- A pinch of ground cloves

Directions:
Heat up a pan over medium heat, add the coconut cream, and heat up for a few minutes. Add the stevia and almonds, stir well, and cook for 5 minutes. Add the cloves, cardamom, nutmeg, and cinnamon and stir well. Transfer to a bowl and serve hot.

Nutrition: Calories - 200, Fat - 12, Fiber - 4, Carbs - 8, Protein - 16

Granola

Preparation time: 10 minutes
Cooking time: 0 minutes
Servings: 2

Ingredients:
- 2 tablespoons chocolate, chopped
- 7 strawberries, hulled, and chopped
- A splash of lemon juice
- 2 tablespoons pecans, chopped

Directions:
In a bowl, mix the chocolate with strawberries, pecans, and lemon juice. Stir well and serve cold.

Nutrition: Calories - 200, Fat - 5, Fiber - 4, Carbs - 7, Protein - 8

Almond Cereal

Preparation time: 5 minutes
Cooking time: 0 minutes.
Servings: 1

Ingredients:
- 2 tablespoons almonds, chopped
- 2 tablespoons sunflower seeds, roasted
- ⅓ cup coconut milk
- 1 tablespoon chia seeds
- ⅓ cup water
- ½ cup blueberries
- 1 small banana, peeled and chopped

Directions:
In a bowl, mix the chia seeds with coconut milk, and set aside for 5 minutes. In a food processor, mix the half of the sunflower seeds with almonds, and pulse them well. Add this to chia seeds mixture. Add the water and stir. Top with the rest of the sunflower seeds, banana pieces, and blueberries and serve.

Nutrition: Calories - 200, Fat - 3, Fiber - 2, Carbs - 5, Protein - 4

Nutty Breakfast Bowl

Preparation time: 5 minutes
Cooking time: 0 minutes
Servings: 1

Ingredients:
- 1 teaspoon pecans, chopped
- 1 cup coconut milk
- 1 teaspoon walnuts, chopped
- 1 teaspoon pistachios, chopped
- 1 teaspoon almonds, chopped
- 1 teaspoon pine nuts, raw
- 1 teaspoon sunflower seeds, raw
- 1 teaspoon raw honey
- 1 teaspoon sunflower seeds, raw
- 2 teaspoons raspberries

Directions:
In a bowl, mix the milk with honey and stir. Add the pecans, walnuts, almonds, pistachios, pine nuts, and sunflower seeds. Stir, top with raspberries, and serve.

Nutrition: Calories - 100, Fat - 2, Fiber - 4, Carbs - 5, Protein - 6

Breakfast Bread

Preparation time: 10 minutes
Cooking time: 3 minutes
Servings: 4

Ingredients:
- ½ teaspoon baking powder
- ⅓ cup almond flour
- 1 egg, whisked
- A pinch of salt
- 2 ½ tablespoons coconut oil

Directions:
Grease a large microwave-safe mug with some of the oil. In a bowl, mix the egg with flour, salt, oil, and baking powder. Pour this into a mug and cook in a microwave for 3 minutes on high. Let the bread to cool, take out of the mug, slice, and serve.

Nutrition: Calories - 132, Fat - 12, Fiber - 1, Carbs - 3, Protein - 4

Breakfast Muffins

Preparation time: 10 minutes
Cooking time: 30 minutes
Servings: 4

Ingredients:
- ½ cup almond milk
- 6 eggs
- 1 tablespoon coconut oil
- Salt and ground black pepper, to taste
- ¼ cup kale, chopped
- 8 prosciutto slices
- ¼ cup fresh chives, chopped

Directions:
In a bowl, mix the eggs with salt, pepper, milk, chives, and kale. Grease a muffin tray with melted coconut oil, line with prosciutto slices, pour the eggs mixture, place in an oven, and bake at 350°F for 30 minutes. Transfer muffins to a platter, and serve.

Nutrition: Calories - 140, Fat - 3, Fiber - 1, Carbs - 3, Protein - 10

Vegetable Breakfast Bread

Preparation time: 10 minutes
Cooking time: 25 minutes
Servings: 7

Ingredients:
- 1 cauliflower head, separated into florets
- ½ cup fresh parsley, chopped
- 1 cup spinach, torn
- 1 onion, peeled and chopped
- 1 tablespoon coconut oil
- ½ cup pecans, ground
- 3 eggs
- 2 garlic cloves, peeled and minced
- Salt and ground black pepper, to taste

Directions:
In a food processor, mix the cauliflower florets with some salt, and pepper, and pulse well. Heat up a pan with the oil over medium heat, add the cauliflower, onion, and garlic, some salt and pepper, stir, and cook for 10 minutes. In a bowl, mix the eggs with salt, pepper, parsley, spinach, and nuts, and stir. Add the cauliflower mixture, and stir well. Spread this mixture into forms placed on a baking sheet, heat oven to 350°F, and bake for 15 minutes. Serve warm.

Nutrition: Calories - 140, Fat - 3, Fiber - 3, Carbs - 4, Protein - 8

Breadless Breakfast Sandwich

Preparation time: 10 minutes
Cooking time: 10 minutes
Servings: 1

Ingredients:
- 2 eggs
- Salt and ground black pepper, to taste
- 2 tablespoons butter
- ¼ pound pork sausage, minced
- ¼ cup water
- 1 tablespoon guacamole

Directions:
In a bowl, mix the minced sausage meat with some salt and pepper, and stir well. Shape a patty from this mixture and place it on a working surface. Heat up a pan with 1 tablespoon butter over medium heat, add the sausage patty, fry for 3 minutes on each side, and transfer to a plate. Crack an egg into 2 bowls and whisk them with some salt and pepper. Heat up a pan with the rest of the butter over medium-high heat, place 2 biscuit cutters that you've greased with some butter in the pan and add an egg to each one. Add the water to the pan, reduce heat, cover pan, and cook eggs for 3 minutes. Transfer these egg "buns" to paper towels and drain the excess grease. Place sausage patty on one egg "bun," spread guacamole over it, and top with the other egg "bun,"

Nutrition: Calories - 200, Fat - 4, Fiber - 6, Carbs - 5, Protein - 10

Chicken Breakfast Muffins

Preparation time: 10 minutes
Cooking time: 1 hour
Servings: 3

Ingredients:
- ¾ pound chicken breast, boneless
- Salt and ground black pepper, to taste
- ½ teaspoon garlic powder
- 3 tablespoons hot sauce mixed with 3 tablespoons melted coconut oil
- 6 eggs
- 2 tablespoons green onions, chopped

Directions:
Season the chicken breast with salt, pepper, and garlic powder, place it on a lined baking sheet, and bake in the oven at 425°F for 25 minutes. Transfer the chicken breast to a bowl, shred with a fork, and mix with half of the hot sauce and melted coconut oil. Toss to coat, and set aside. In a bowl, mix the eggs with salt, pepper, green onions, and the rest of the hot sauce mixed with oil and whisk. Divide this mixture into a muffin tray, top each with shredded chicken, place in an oven at 350°F, and bake for 30 minutes. Serve the muffins hot.

Nutrition: Calories - 140, Fat - 8, Fiber - 1, Carbs - 2, Protein - 13

Herbed Biscuits

Preparation time: 10 minutes
Cooking time: 15 minutes
Servings: 6

Ingredients:
- 6 tablespoons coconut oil
- 6 tablespoons coconut flour
- 2 garlic cloves, peeled and minced
- ¼ cup onion, minced
- 2 eggs
- Salt and ground black pepper, to taste
- 1 tablespoons fresh parsley, chopped
- 2 tablespoons coconut milk
- ½ teaspoon apple cider vinegar
- ¼ teaspoon baking soda

Directions:
In a bowl, mix the coconut flour with eggs, oil, garlic, onion, coconut milk, parsley, salt, and pepper, and stir well. In a bowl, mix the vinegar with baking soda, stir well, and add to the batter. Drop spoonfuls of this batter on lined baking sheets and shape into circles. Place in an oven at 350°F and bake for 15 minutes. Serve hot.

Nutrition: Calories - 140, Fat - 6, Fiber - 2, Carbs - 10, Protein - 12

Avocado Muffins

Preparation time: 10 minutes
Cooking time: 20 minutes
Servings: 12

Ingredients:
- 4 eggs
- 6 bacon slices, chopped
- 1 onion, peeled and chopped
- 1 cup coconut milk
- 2 cups avocado, pitted, peeled, and chopped
- Salt and ground black pepper, to taste
- ½ teaspoon baking soda
- ½ cup coconut flour

Directions:
Heat up a pan over medium heat, add the onion, and bacon, stir, and cook for a few minutes. In a bowl, mash avocado pieces with a fork and whisk with the eggs. Add the milk, salt, pepper, baking soda, and coconut flour, and stir. Add the bacon mixture, and stir again. Grease a muffin tray with the coconut oil, divide the eggs and avocado mixture into the tray, place in an oven at 350ºF, and bake for 20 minutes. Divide the muffins on plates, and serve them.

Nutrition: Calories - 200, Fat - 7, Fiber - 4, Carbs - 7, Protein - 5

Bacon and Lemon Thyme Muffins

Preparation time: 10 minutes
Cooking time: 20 minutes
Servings: 12

Ingredients:
- 1 cup bacon, diced
- Salt and ground black pepper, to taste
- ½ cup butter, melted
- 3 cups almond flour
- 1 teaspoon baking soda
- 4 eggs
- 2 teaspoons lemon thyme

Directions:
In a bowl, mix the flour with baking soda, and eggs, and stir well. Add the butter, lemon thyme, bacon, salt, and pepper, and whisk. Divide this mixture into a lined muffin pan, place in an oven at 350ºF, and bake for 20 minutes. Let the muffins to cool, divide on plates, and serve.

Nutrition: Calories - 213, Fat - 7, Fiber - 2, Carbs - 9, Protein - 8

Cheese and Oregano Muffins

Preparation time: 10 minutes
Cooking time: 25 minutes
Servings: 6

Ingredients:
- 2 tablespoons olive oil
- 1 egg
- 2 tablespoons Parmesan cheese
- ½ teaspoon dried oregano
- 1 cup almond flour
- ¼ teaspoon baking soda
- Salt and ground black pepper, to taste
- ½ cup coconut milk
- 1 cup cheddar cheese, grated

Directions:
In a bowl, mix the flour with oregano, salt, pepper, Parmesan cheese, and baking soda. In another bowl, mix the coconut milk with egg, and olive oil, and stir well. Combine the 2 mixtures, and whisk. Add the cheddar cheese, stir, pour the mixture into a lined muffin tray, and place in an oven at 350ºF for 25 minutes. Let the muffins cool for a few minutes and serve.

Nutrition: Calories - 160, Fat - 3, Fiber - 2, Carbs - 6, Protein - 10

Turkey Breakfast

Preparation time: 10 minutes
Cooking time: 20 minutes
Servings: 1

Ingredients:
- 2 avocado slices
- Salt and ground black pepper, to taste
- 2 bacon sliced
- 2 turkey breast slices, already cooked
- 2 tablespoons coconut oil
- 2 eggs, whisked

Directions:
Heat up a pan over medium heat, add the bacon slices, and brown them for a few minutes. Heat up another pan with the oil over medium heat, add the eggs, salt, and pepper, and scramble them. Divide the turkey breast slices, scrambled eggs, bacon slices, and avocado slices on 2 plates and serve.

Nutrition: Calories - 135, Fat - 7, Fiber - 2, Carbs - 4, Protein - 10

Burrito

Preparation time: 10 minutes
Cooking time: 16 minutes
Servings: 1

Ingredients:
- 1 teaspoon coconut oil
- 1 teaspoon garlic powder
- 1 teaspoon cumin
- ¼ pound ground beef
- 1 teaspoon sweet paprika
- 1 teaspoon onion powder
- 1 onion, peeled, and julienned
- 1 teaspoon fresh cilantro, chopped
- Salt and ground black pepper, to taste
- 3 eggs

Directions:
Heat up a pan over medium heat, add the beef, and brown for a few minutes. Add the salt, pepper, cumin, garlic, and onion powder, and paprika, stir, cook for 4 minutes, and take off the heat. In a bowl, mix the eggs with salt, and pepper, and whisk. Heat up a pan with the oil over medium heat, add the egg, spread evenly, and cook for 6 minutes. Transfer the egg burrito to a plate, divide the beef mixture, add the onion, and cilantro, roll, and serve.

Nutrition: Calories - 280, Fat - 12, Fiber - 4, Carbs - 7, Protein - 14

Breakfast Hash

Preparation time: 10 minutes
Cooking time: 16 minutes
Servings: 2

Ingredients:
- 1 tablespoon coconut oil
- 2 garlic cloves, peeled and minced
- ½ cup beef stock
- Salt and ground black pepper, to taste
- 1 onion, peeled and chopped
- 2 cups corned beef, chopped
- 1 pound radishes, cut in quarters

Directions:
Heat up a pan with the oil over medium-high heat, add the onion, stir, and cook for 4 minutes. Add the radishes, stir, and cook for 5 minutes. Add the garlic, stir, and cook for 1 minute. Add the stock, beef, salt, and pepper, stir, cook for 5 minutes, take off the heat, and serve.

Nutrition: Calories - 240, Fat - 7, Fiber - 3, Carbs - 12, Protein - 8

Brussels Sprout Delight

Preparation time: 10 minutes
Cooking time: 12 minutes
Servings: 3

Ingredients:
- 3 eggs
- Salt and ground black pepper, to taste
- 1 tablespoon butter, melted
- 2 shallots, peeled and minced
- 2 garlic cloves, peeled and minced
- 12 ounces Brussels sprouts, sliced thin
- 2 ounces bacon, chopped
- 1½ tablespoons apple cider vinegar

Directions:
Heat up a pan over medium heat, add the bacon, stir, cook until crispy, transfer to a plate, and set aside. Heat up the pan again over medium heat, add the shallots and garlic, stir, and cook for 30 seconds. Add the Brussels sprouts, salt, pepper, and apple cider vinegar, stir, and cook for 5 minutes. Return the bacon to pan, stir, and cook for 5 minutes. Add the butter, stir, and make a hole in the center. Crack the eggs into the pan, cook until they are done, and serve.

Nutrition: Calories - 240, Fat - 7, Fiber - 4, Carbs - 7, Protein - 12

Cereal Nibs

Preparation time: 10 minutes
Cooking time: 45 minutes
Servings: 4

Ingredients:
- 4 tablespoons hemp hearts
- ½ cup chia seeds
- 1 cup water
- 1 tablespoon vanilla extract
- 1 tablespoon psyllium powder
- 2 tablespoons coconut oil
- 1 tablespoon swerve
- 2 tablespoons cocoa nibs

Directions:
In a bowl, mix the chia seeds with water, stir, and set aside for 5 minutes. Add the hemp hearts, vanilla extract, psyllium powder, oil, and swerve and stir well with a mixer. Add the cocoa nibs and stir until you obtain a dough. Divide the dough into 2 pieces, shape into cylinder form, place on a lined baking sheet, flatten well, cover with a parchment paper, place in an oven at 285ºF, and bake for 20 minutes. Remove the parchment paper, and bake for 25 minutes. Take the cylinders out of the oven, set aside to cool down, and cut into small pieces before serving.

Nutrition: Calories - 245, Fat - 12, Fiber - 12, Carbs - 2, Protein - 9

Chia Pudding

Preparation time: 10 minutes
Cooking time: 30 minutes
Servings: 2

Ingredients:
- 2 tablespoons coffee
- 2 cups water
- ⅓ cup chia seeds
- 1 tablespoon swerve
- 1 tablespoon vanilla extract
- 2 tablespoons cocoa nibs
- ⅓ cup coconut cream

Directions:
Heat up a small pot with the water over medium heat, bring to a boil, add the coffee, simmer for 15 minutes, take off the heat, and strain into a bowl. Add the vanilla extract, coconut cream, swerve, cocoa nibs, and chia seeds, stir well, keep in the refrigerator for 30 minutes, divide into 2 breakfast bowls, and serve.

Nutrition: Calories - 100, Fat - 0. 4, Fiber - 4, Carbs - 3, Protein - 3

Hemp Porridge

Preparation time: 3 minutes
Cooking time: 3 minutes
Servings: 1

Ingredients:
- 1 tablespoon chia seeds
- 1 cup almond milk
- 2 tablespoons flaxseeds
- ½ cup hemp hearts
- ½ teaspoon ground cinnamon
- 1 tablespoon stevia
- ¾ teaspoon vanilla extract
- ¼ cup almond flour
- 1 tablespoon hemp hearts, for serving

Directions:
In a pan, mix almond milk with ½ cup hemp hearts, chia seeds, stevia, flaxseeds, cinnamon, and vanilla extract, stir well, and heat up over medium heat. Cook for 2 minutes, take off the heat, add the almond flour, stir well, and pour into a bowl. Top with 1 tablespoon hemp hearts, and serve.

Nutrition: Calories - 230, Fat - 12, Fiber - 7, Carbs - 3, Protein - 43

Simple Breakfast Cereal

Preparation time: 10 minutes
Cooking time: 3 minutes
Servings: 2

Ingredients:
- ½ cup coconut, shredded
- 4 teaspoons butter
- 2 cups almond milk
- 1 tablespoon stevia
- A pinch of salt
- ⅓ cup macadamia nuts, chopped
- ⅓ cup walnuts, chopped
- ⅓ cup flaxseed

Directions:
Heat up a pot with the butter over medium heat, add the milk, coconut, salt, macadamia nuts, walnuts, flaxseed, and stevia, and stir well. Cook for 3 minutes, stir again, take off the heat, and set aside for 10 minutes. Divide into 2 bowls, and serve.

Nutrition: Calories - 140, Fat - 3, Fiber - 2, Carbs - 1. 5, Protein - 7

Simple Egg Porridge

Preparation time: 10 minutes
Cooking time: 4 minutes
Servings: 2

Ingredients:
- 2 eggs
- 1 tablespoon stevia
- ⅓ cup heavy cream
- 2 tablespoons butter, melted
- A pinch of ground cinnamon

Directions:
In a bowl, mix the eggs with stevia and heavy cream, and whisk. Heat up a pan with the butter over medium-high heat, add the egg mixture, and cook until they are done. Transfer to 2 bowls, sprinkle cinnamon on top, and serve.

Nutrition: Calories - 340, Fat - 12, Fiber - 10, Carbs - 3, Protein - 14

Pancakes

Preparation time: 3 minutes
Cooking time: 12 minutes
Servings: 4

Ingredients:
- ½ teaspoon ground cinnamon
- 1 teaspoon stevia
- 2 eggs
- Vegetable oil cooking spray
- 2 ounces cream cheese

Directions:
In a blender, mix eggs with cream cheese, stevia, and cinnamon, and blend well. Heat up a pan with some cooking spray over medium-high heat, pour ¼ of the batter, spread well, cook for 2 minutes, flip, and cook for 1 minute. Transfer to a plate, and repeat with the rest of the batter. Serve warm.

Nutrition: Calories - 344, Fat - 23, Fiber - 12, Carbs - 3, Protein - 16

Almond Pancakes

Preparation time: 10 minutes
Cooking time: 10 minutes
Servings: 12

Ingredients:
- 6 eggs
- A pinch of salt
- ½ cup coconut flour
- ¼ cup stevia
- ⅓ cup coconut, shredded
- ½ teaspoon baking powder
- 1 cup almond milk
- ¼ cup coconut oil
- 1 teaspoon almond extract
- ¼ cup almonds, toasted
- 2 ounces cocoa powder
- Vegetable oil cooking spray

Directions:
In a bowl, mix the coconut flour with stevia, salt, baking powder, and coconut, and stir. Add the coconut oil, eggs, almond milk, and almond extract, and stir well. Add the cocoa powder and almonds, and whisk again. Heat up a pan with cooking spray over medium heat, add 2 tablespoons batter, spread into a circle, cook until it's golden, flip, cook again until done, and transfer to a plate in a warm oven. Repeat with the rest of the batter and serve right away.

Nutrition: Calories - 266, Fat - 13, Fiber - 8, Carbs - 10, Protein - 11

Pumpkin Pancakes

Preparation time: 10 minutes
Cooking time: 15 minutes
Servings: 6

Ingredients:
- 1 ounce egg white protein
- 2 ounces hazelnut flour
- 2 ounces flaxseeds, ground
- 1 teaspoon baking powder
- 1 cup coconut cream
- 1 tablespoon chai masala
- 1 teaspoon vanilla extract
- ½ cup pumpkin puree
- 3 eggs
- 5 drops stevia
- 1 tablespoon swerve
- 1 teaspoon coconut oil

Directions:
In a bowl, mix the flaxseeds with hazelnut flour, egg white protein, baking powder, and chai masala, and stir. In another bowl, mix the coconut cream with vanilla extract, pumpkin puree, eggs, stevia, and swerve, and stir. Combine the 2 mixtures and stir well. Heat up a pan with the oil over medium-high heat, pour 1/6 of the batter, spread into a circle, cover, reduce heat to low, cook for 3 minutes on each side, and transfer to a plate.
Keep warm, repeat with the rest of the batter, and serve right away.

Nutrition: Calories - 400, Fat - 23, Fiber - 4, Carbs - 5, Protein - 21

Simple French Toast

Preparation time: 5 minutes
Cooking time: 45 minutes
Servings: 18

Ingredients:
- 1 cup whey protein
- 12 egg whites
- 4 ounces cream cheese

For the French toast:
- 1 teaspoon vanilla extract
- ½ cup coconut milk
- 2 eggs
- 1 teaspoon ground cinnamon
- ½ cup butter, melted
- ½ cup almond milk
- ½ cup swerve

Directions:
In a bowl, mix the 12 egg whites with a mixer for a few minutes. Add the protein and stir gently. Add the cream cheese and stir again. Pour this into 2 greased bread pans, place in an oven at 325ºF, and bake for 45 minutes. Let the bread to cool down, and slice into 18 pieces. In a bowl, mix the 2 eggs with vanilla extract, cinnamon, and coconut milk, and whisk. Dip bread slices in this mixture. Heat up a pan with some coconut oil over medium heat, add the bread slices, cook until they are golden on each side, and divide on plates. Heat up a pan with the butter over high heat, add the almond milk, and heat up. Add the swerve, stir, and take off the heat.
Leave aside to cool, and drizzle over French toast slices.

Nutrition: Calories - 200, Fat - 12, Fiber - 1, Carbs - 1, Protein - 7

Waffles

Preparation time: 10 minutes
Cooking time: 20 minutes
Servings: 5

Ingredients:
- 5 eggs, separated
- 3 tablespoons almond milk
- 1 teaspoon baking powder
- 3 tablespoons stevia
- 4 tablespoons coconut flour
- 2 teaspoon vanilla extract
- 4 ounces butter, melted

Directions:
In a bowl, whisk the egg whites using a mixer. In another bowl, mix the flour with stevia, baking powder, and egg yolks, and whisk. Add the vanilla extract, butter, and milk, and stir well. Add the egg whites and stir. Pour some of the mixture into a waffle maker, and cook until it's golden. Repeat with the rest of the batter, and serve the waffles right away.

Nutrition: Calories - 240, Fat - 23, Fiber - 2, Carbs - 4, Protein - 7

Baked Granola

Preparation time: 10 minutes
Cooking time: 60 minutes
Servings: 4

Ingredients:
- ½ cup almonds, chopped
- 1 cup pecans, chopped
- ½ cup walnuts, chopped
- ½ cup coconut, flaked
- ¼ cup flax meal
- ½ cup almond milk
- ¼ cup sunflower seeds
- ¼ cup sunflower seeds
- ½ cup stevia
- ¼ cup butter, melted
- 1 teaspoon honey
- 1 teaspoon vanilla extract
- 1 teaspoon ground cinnamon
- A pinch of salt
- ½ teaspoon ground nutmeg
- ¼ cup water

Directions:
In a bowl, mix the almonds with pecans, walnuts, coconut, flax meal, milk, sunflower seeds, sunflower seeds, stevia, butter, honey, vanilla extract, cinnamon, salt, nutmeg, and water, and whisk. Grease a baking sheet with parchment paper, spread granola mixture, and press well. Cover with another piece of parchment paper, place in an oven at 250ºF, and bake for 1 hour. Take the granola out of the oven, set aside to cool down, break into pieces, and serve.

Nutrition: Calories - 340, Fat - 32, Fiber - 12, Carbs - 20, Protein - 20

Nutty Breakfast Smoothie

Preparation time: 5 minutes
Cooking time: 0 minutes
Servings: 1

Ingredients:
- 2 brazil nuts
- 1 cup coconut milk
- 10 almonds
- 2 cups spinach leaves
- 1 teaspoon greens powder
- 1 teaspoon whey protein
- 1 tablespoon psyllium seeds
- 1 tablespoon potato starch

Directions:
In a blender, mix the spinach with Brazil nuts, coconut milk, and almonds and blend well. Add the green powder, whey protein, potato starch, and psyllium seeds, and blend well. Pour into a tall glass and serve.

Nutrition: Calories - 340, Fat - 30, Fiber - 7, Carbs - 7, Protein - 12

Kiwi and Pineapple Smoothie

Preparation time: 5 minutes
Cooking time: 0 minutes
Servings: 6

Ingredients:
- 1 cup lettuce leaves
- 4 cups water
- 2 tablespoons fresh parsley
- 1 tablespoon fresh ginger, grated
- 1 tablespoon swerve
- 1 cup cucumber, sliced
- ½ avocado, pitted and peeled
- ½ cup kiwi, peeled and sliced
- ⅓ cup pineapple, chopped

Directions:
In a blender, mix the water with lettuce leaves, pineapple, parsley, cucumber, ginger, kiwi, avocado, and swerve, and blend well. Pour into glasses and serve.

Nutrition: Calories - 60, Fat - 2, Fiber - 3, Carbs - 3, Protein - 1

Breakfast in a Glass

Preparation time: 3 minutes
Cooking time: 0 minutes
Servings: 2

Ingredients:
- 10 ounces canned coconut milk
- 1 cup greens
- ¼ cup cocoa nibs
- 1 cup water
- 1 cup cherries, frozen
- ¼ cup cocoa powder
- 1 small avocado, pitted and peeled
- ¼ teaspoon turmeric

Directions:
In a blender, mix the coconut milk with avocado, cocoa powder, cherries, and turmeric and blend well. Add the water, greens, and cocoa nibs, blend for 2 minutes, pour into glasses, and serve.

Nutrition: Calories - 100, Fat - 3, Fiber - 2, Carbs - 3, Protein - 5

Steak and Eggs

Preparation time: 10 minutes
Cooking time: 10 minutes
Servings: 1

Ingredients:
- 4 ounces sirloin steak
- 1 small avocado, pitted, peeled, and sliced
- 3 eggs
- 1 tablespoon butter
- Salt and ground black pepper, to taste

Directions:
Heat up a pan with the butter over medium-high heat, crack eggs into the pan, and cook them as you wish. Season with salt and pepper, take off the heat, and transfer to a plate. Heat up another pan over medium-high heat, add the steak, cook for 4 minutes, take off the heat, set aside to cool down, and cut into thin strips. Season with some salt and pepper and place next to the eggs. Add the avocado slices on the side and serve.

Nutrition: Calories - 500, Fat - 34, Fiber - 10, Carbs - 3, Protein - 40

Chicken Quiche

Preparation time: 10 minutes
Cooking time: 45 minutes
Servings: 5

Ingredients:
- 7 eggs
- 2 cups almond flour
- 2 tablespoons coconut oil
- Salt and ground black pepper, to taste
- 2 zucchini, grated
- ½ cup heavy cream
- 1 teaspoon fennel seeds
- 1 teaspoon dried oregano
- 1 pound ground chicken

Directions:
In a food processor, blend the almond flour with a pinch of salt. Add the 1 egg and coconut oil and blend well. Place dough in a greased pie pan and press well on the bottom. Heat up a pan over medium heat, add the chicken, brown for a couple of minutes, take off the heat, and leave aside. In a bowl, mix the 6 eggs with salt, pepper, oregano, cream, and fennel seeds, and whisk. Add the chicken and stir again. Pour this into pie crust, spread, place in an oven at 350ºF, and bake for 40 minutes. Let the pie to cool before slicing and serving.

Nutrition: Calories - 300, Fat - 23, Fiber - 3, Carbs - 4, Protein - 18

Chicken Omelet

Preparation time: 10 minutes
Cooking time: 10 minutes
Servings: 1

Ingredients:
- 1 ounce rotisserie chicken, shredded
- 1 teaspoon mustard
- 1 tablespoon mayonnaise
- 1 tomato, cored and chopped
- 2 bacon slices, cooked and crumbled
- 2 eggs
- 1 small avocado, pitted, peeled, and chopped
- Salt and ground black pepper, to taste

Directions:
In a bowl, mix the eggs with some salt and pepper and whisk. Heat up a pan over medium heat, spray with some cooking oil, add the eggs, and cook the omelet for 5 minutes. Add the chicken, avocado, tomato, bacon, mayonnaise, and mustard on one half of the omelet. Fold the omelet, cover pan, and cook for 5 minutes. Transfer to a plate and serve.

Nutrition: Calories - 400, Fat - 32, Fiber - 6, Carbs - 4, Protein - 25

Simple Smoothie Bowl

Preparation time: 5 minutes
Cooking time: 0 minutes
Servings: 1

Ingredients:
- 2 ice cubes
- 1 tablespoon coconut oil
- 2 tablespoons heavy cream
- 1 cup spinach
- ½ cup almond milk
- 1 teaspoon protein powder
- 4 raspberries
- 1 tablespoon coconut, shredded
- 4 walnuts
- 1 teaspoon chia seeds

Directions:
In a blender, mix the milk with the spinach, cream, ice, protein powder, and coconut oil, blend well, and transfer to a bowl. Top the bowl with raspberries, coconut, walnuts, and chia seeds and serve.

Nutrition: Calories - 450, Fat - 34, Fiber - 4, Carbs - 4, Protein - 35

Feta Omelet

Preparation time: 10 minutes
Cooking time: 10 minutes
Servings: 1

Ingredients:
- 3 eggs
- 1 tablespoon butter
- 1 ounce feta cheese, crumbled
- 1 tablespoon heavy cream
- 1 tablespoon jarred pesto
- Salt and ground black pepper, to taste

Directions:
In a bowl, mix the eggs with heavy cream, salt, and pepper, and whisk. Heat up a pan with the butter over medium-high heat, add the whisked eggs, spread into the pan, and cook the omelet until it's fluffy. Sprinkle the cheese and spread pesto on the omelet, fold in half, cover pan, and cook for 5 minutes. Transfer the omelet to a plate and serve.

Nutrition: Calories - 500, Fat - 43, Fiber - 6, Carbs - 3, Protein - 30

Breakfast Meatloaf

Preparation time: 10 minutes
Cooking time: 35 minutes
Servings: 4

Ingredients:
- 1 teaspoon butter
- 1 onion, peeled and chopped
- 1 pound sweet sausage, chopped
- 6 eggs
- 1 cup cheddar cheese, shredded
- 4 ounces cream cheese, softened
- Salt and ground black pepper, to taste
- 2 tablespoons scallions, chopped

Directions:
In a bowl, mix the eggs with salt, pepper, onion, sausage, and half of the cream, and whisk. Grease a loaf pan with the butter, pour sausage, and eggs mixture, place in an oven at 350ºF, and bake for 30 minutes. Take the meatloaf out of the oven, set aside for a couple of minutes, spread the rest of the cream cheese on top, and sprinkle the scallions and cheddar cheese all over. Place meatloaf in the oven again and bake for 5 minutes. Then, place the meatloaf under a broiler for 3 minutes, let it cool, then slice it and serve.

Nutrition: Calories - 560, Fat - 32, Fiber - 1, Carbs - 6, Protein - 45

Breakfast Tuna Salad

Preparation time: 10 minutes
Cooking time: 0 minutes
Servings: 4

Ingredients:
- 2 tablespoons sour cream
- 12 ounces canned tuna in olive oil
- 4 leeks, diced
- Salt and ground black pepper, to taste
- A pinch of red chili flakes
- 1 tablespoon capers
- 8 tablespoons mayonnaise

Directions:
In a salad bowl, mix the tuna with capers, salt, pepper, leeks, chili flakes, sour cream, and mayonnaise. Stir well and serve.

Nutrition: Calories - 160, Fat - 2, Fiber - 1, Carbs - 2, Protein - 6

Breakfast Salad in a Jar

Preparation time: 10 minutes
Cooking time: 0 minutes
Servings: 1

Ingredients:
- 1 ounce greens
- 1 ounce red bell pepper, seeded and chopped
- 1 ounce cherry tomatoes, halved
- 4 ounces rotisserie chicken, chopped
- 4 tablespoons extra virgin olive oil
- ½ scallion, chopped
- 1 ounce cucumber, chopped
- Salt and ground black pepper, to taste

Directions:
In a bowl, mix the greens with the bell pepper, tomatoes, scallion, cucumber, salt, pepper, and olive oil and toss to coat well. Transfer this to a jar, top with chicken pieces, and serve.

Nutrition: Calories - 180, Fat - 12, Fiber - 4, Carbs - 5, Protein - 17

Naan Bread and Butter

Preparation time: 10 minutes
Cooking time: 10 minutes
Servings: 6

Ingredients:
- 7 tablespoons coconut oil
- ¾ cup coconut flour
- 2 tablespoons psyllium powder
- ½ teaspoon baking powder
- Salt, to taste
- 2 cups hot water
- Some coconut oil, for frying
- 2 garlic cloves, peeled and minced
- 3. 5 ounces butter

Directions:
In a bowl, mix the coconut flour with baking powder, salt, and psyllium powder, and stir. Add the coconut oil and the hot water and knead the dough. Set aside for 5 minutes, divide into 6 balls, and flatten them on a working surface. Heat up a pan with some coconut oil over medium-high heat, add the naan bread to the pan, fry them until golden brown, and transfer them to a plate. Heat up a pan with the butter over medium-high heat, add the garlic, salt, and pepper, stir, and cook for 2 minutes. Brush the naan bread with this mixture, and pour the rest into a bowl and serve.

Nutrition: Calories - 140, Fat - 9, Fiber - 2, Carbs - 3, Protein - 4

Ketogenic Recipes for Lunch

Lunch Caesar Salad

Preparation time: 10 minutes
Cooking time: 0 minutes
Servings: 2

Ingredients:
- 1 avocado, pitted, peeled, and sliced
- Salt and ground black pepper, to taste
- 3 tablespoons creamy Caesar dressing
- 1 cup bacon, cooked and crumbled
- 1 chicken breast, grilled and shredded

Directions:
In a salad bowl, mix the avocado with bacon and chicken breast, and stir. Add the dressing, salt, and pepper, toss to coat, divide into 2 bowls, and serve.

Nutrition: Calories - 334, Fat - 23, Fiber - 4, Carbs - 3, Protein - 18

Lunch Tacos

Preparation time: 10 minutes
Cooking time: 25 minutes
Servings: 3

Ingredients:
- 2 cups cheddar cheese, grated
- 1 small avocado, pitted, peeled, and chopped
- 1 cup taco meat, cooked
- 2 teaspoons sriracha sauce
- ¼ cup tomatoes, cored and chopped
- Vegetable oil cooking spray
- Salt and ground black pepper, to taste

Directions:
Spray some cooking oil on lined baking dish. Spread the cheddar cheese on the baking sheet, place in an oven at 400°F, and bake for 15 minutes. Spread taco meat over cheese, and bake for 10 minutes. In a bowl, mix the avocado with tomatoes, sriracha sauce, salt, and pepper, and stir. Spread this over the taco and cheddar layers, let the tacos to cool, slice using a pizza cutter, and serve.

Nutrition: Calories - 400, Fat - 23, Fiber - 0, Carbs - 2, Protein - 37

Lunch Pizza

Preparation time: 10 minutes
Cooking time: 7 minutes
Servings: 4

Ingredients:
- 1 tablespoon olive oil
- 2 tablespoons butter
- 2 cups mozzarella cheese, shredded
- ¼ cup mascarpone cheese
- 1 tablespoon heavy cream
- 1 teaspoon garlic, minced
- Salt and ground black pepper, to taste
- A pinch of lemon pepper
- ⅓ cup broccoli florets, steamed
- Some Asiago cheese, shaved, for serving

Directions:
Heat up a pan with the oil over medium heat, add the pizza cheese mixture, and spread into a circle. Add the mozzarella cheese, and spread it into a circle too. Cook everything for 5 minutes, and transfer to a plate. Heat up the pan with the butter over medium heat, add the mascarpone cheese, cream, salt, pepper, lemon pepper, and garlic, stir, and cook for 5 minutes. Drizzle half of this mixture over cheese crust. Add the broccoli florets to the pan with the rest of the mascarpone mixture, stir, and cook for 1 minute. Add this on top of the pizza, sprinkle with Asiago cheese at the end, and serve.

Nutrition: Calories - 250, Fat - 15, Fiber - 1, Carbs - 3, Protein - 10

Pizza Rolls

Preparation time: 10 minutes
Cooking time: 30 minutes
Servings: 6

Ingredients:
- ¼ cup mixed red and green bell peppers, seeded and chopped
- 2 cup mozzarella cheese, shredded
- 1 teaspoon pizza seasoning
- 2 tablespoons onion, peeled and chopped
- 1 tomato, cored and chopped
- Salt and ground black pepper, to taste
- ¼ cup pizza sauce
- ½ cup sausage, crumbled and cooked

Directions:
Spread the mozzarella cheese on a lined and lightly greased baking sheet, sprinkle pizza seasoning on top, place in an oven at 400°F, and bake for 20 minutes. Take the pizza crust out of the oven, spread the sausage, onion, bell peppers, and tomatoes all over, and drizzle the tomato sauce on top. Place in an oven again, and bake for 10 minutes. Take pizza out of the oven, set aside for a couple of minutes, slice into 6 pieces, roll each piece, and serve.

Nutrition: Calories - 117, Fat - 7, Fiber - 1, Carbs - 2, Protein - 11

Cheese Dough Pizza

Preparation time: 10 minutes
Cooking time: 15 minutes
Servings: 2

Ingredients:
- 1½ cups cheddar cheese, shredded
- 1½ cups cheese blend
- 2 beef hot dogs, diced
- A drizzle of olive oil
- 1 pound ground beef
- Salt and ground black pepper, to taste
- ¼ teaspoon paprika
- ¼ teaspoon Old Bay Seasoning
- ¼ teaspoon onion powder
- ¼ teaspoon garlic powder
- 1 cup lettuce leaves, chopped
- 1 tablespoon Thousand Island dressing
- 2 tablespoons dill pickles, chopped
- 2 tablespoons onion, peeled and chopped
- ½ cup American cheese, shredded
- Some ketchup, for serving
- Some mustard, for serving

Directions:
Heat up a pan with a drizzle of oil over medium heat, add the half of the cheese blend, spread into a circle, and top with half of the cheddar cheese. Spread this into a circle, cook for 5 minutes, transfer to a cutting board, and set aside for a few minutes to cool down. Heat up the pan again, add the rest of the cheese blend, and spread into a circle. Add the rest of the cheddar, also spread out in a circle, cook for 5 minutes, and transfer to a cutting board. Spread the Thousand Island dressing over the 2 pizza crusts. Heat up the same pan again over medium heat, add the beef, stir, and brown for a few minutes. Add the salt, pepper, Old Bay Seasoning, paprika, onion powder, and garlic powder, stir, and cook for a few minutes. Add the hot dog pieces, stir, and cook for 5 minutes. Spread the lettuce, pickles, American cheese, and onions on the 2 pizza crusts. Divide the beef and hot dog mixture, drizzle with mustard and ketchup at the end, and serve.

Nutrition: Calories - 200, Fat - 6, Fiber - 3, Carbs - 1. 5, Protein - 10

Taco Salad

Preparation time: 10 minutes
Cooking time: 20 minutes
Servings: 4

Ingredients:
- ¼ cup fresh cilantro, chopped
- 2 avocados, pitted, peeled, and cut into chunks
- 1 tablespoon lime juice
- ¼ cup white onion, peeled and chopped
- 1 teaspoon garlic, minced
- Salt and ground black pepper, to taste
- 6 cherry tomatoes, cut in quarters
- ½ cup water
- 2-pound ground beef
- 2 cups sour cream
- ¼ cup taco seasoning
- 2 cups lettuce leaves, shredded
- Hot pepper sauce, for serving
- 2 cups cheddar cheese, shredded

Directions:
In a bowl, mix the cilantro with lime juice, avocado, onion, tomatoes, salt, pepper, and garlic, stir well, and set aside in the refrigerator. Heat up a pan over medium heat, add the beef, stir, and brown for 10 minutes. Add the taco seasoning and water, stir, and cook over medium-low heat for 10 minutes. Divide this mixture into 4 serving bowls. Add the sour cream, avocado mixture, lettuce pieces, and cheddar cheese. Drizzle with the cayenne pepper sauce at the end and serve.

Nutrition: Calories - 340, Fat - 30, Fiber - 5, Carbs - 3, Protein - 32

Stuffed Peppers

Preparation time: 10 minutes
Cooking time: 40 minutes
Servings: 4

Ingredients:
- 4 big banana peppers, peeled, tops cut off, and cut into half lengthwise
- 1 tablespoon butter
- Salt and ground black pepper, to taste
- ½ teaspoon herbs de Provence
- 1 pound sweet sausage, chopped
- 3 tablespoons onions, peeled and chopped
- Marinara sauce
- A drizzle of olive oil

Directions:
Season the banana peppers with salt and pepper, drizzle the oil, rub well, and bake in the oven at 350ºF for 20 minutes. Heat up a pan over medium heat, add the sausage pieces, stir, and cook for 5 minutes. Add the onion, herbs de Provence, salt, pepper, and butter, stir well, and cook for 5 minutes. Take the peppers out of the oven, fill them with the sausage mixture, place them in an oven-proof dish, drizzle marinara sauce over them, place in an oven again, and bake for 10 minutes. Serve hot.

Nutrition: Calories - 320, Fat - 8, Fiber - 4, Carbs - 3, Protein - 10

Beef Brisket Burgers

Preparation time: 10 minutes
Cooking time: 25 minutes
Servings: 8

Ingredients:
- 1 pound ground beef brisket
- 1 pound ground beef
- Salt and ground black pepper, to taste
- ½ cup butter
- 1 tablespoon garlic, minced
- 1 tablespoon Italian seasoning
- 2 tablespoons mayonnaise
- 1 tablespoon butter
- 2 tablespoons olive oil
- 1 onion, peeled and chopped
- 1 tablespoon water

Directions:
In a bowl, mix the brisket with ground beef, salt, pepper, Italian seasoning, garlic, and mayonnaise, and stir well. Shape 8 patties and make a pocket in each. Stuff each burger with a butter slice and seal. Heat up a pan with the olive oil over medium heat, add the onions, stir, and cook for 2 minutes. Add the water, stir, and gather them in the corner of the pan. Place the burgers in the pan with the onions and cook them over medium-low heat for 10 minutes. Flip them, add the butter, and cook them for 10 minutes. Divide the burgers on buns and serve them with caramelized onions on top.

Nutrition: Calories - 180, Fat - 8, Fiber - 1, Carbs - 4, Protein - 20

Chili Pepper Burger

Preparation time: 10 minutes
Cooking time: 30 minutes
Servings: 4

Ingredients:

For the sauce:
- 4 chili peppers, chopped
- 1 cup water
- 1 cup almond butter
- 1 teaspoon swerve
- 6 tablespoons coconut aminos
- 4 garlic cloves, peeled and minced
- 1 tablespoon rice vinegar

For the burgers:
- 4 pepper jack cheese slices
- 1½ pounds ground beef
- 1 onion, peeled and sliced
- 8 bacon slices
- 8 lettuce leaves
- Salt and ground black pepper, to taste

Directions:

Heat up a pan with the almond butter over medium heat. Add the water, stir well, and bring to a simmer. Add the coconut aminos and stir well. In a food processor, mix the chili peppers with garlic, swerve, and vinegar, and blend well. Add this to almond butter mixture, stir well, take off the heat, and set aside. In a bowl, mix the beef with salt and pepper, stir, and shape into 4 patties. Place them in a pan, place under a preheated broiler, and broil for 7 minutes. Flip the burgers and broil them for 7 minutes. Place cheese slices on burgers, place under a broiler, and broil for 4 minutes. Heat up a pan over medium heat, add the bacon slices, and fry them for a couple of minutes. Place 2 lettuce leaves on a dish, add the 1 burger on top, then 1 onion slice and 1 bacon slice, and top with some almond butter sauce. Repeat with the rest of the lettuce leaves, burgers, onion, bacon, and sauce.

Nutrition: Calories - 700, Fat - 56, Fiber - 10, Carbs - 7, Protein - 40

Zucchini with Cheese

Preparation time: 10 minutes
Cooking time: 5 minutes
Servings: 1

Ingredients:
- 1 tablespoon olive oil
- 3 tablespoons butter
- 2 cups zucchini, cut with a spiralizer
- 1 teaspoon red pepper flakes
- 1 tablespoon garlic, minced
- 1 tablespoon red bell pepper, seeded and chopped
- Salt and ground black pepper, to taste
- 1 tablespoon fresh basil, chopped
- ¼ cup Asiago cheese, shaved
- ¼ cup Parmesan cheese, grated

Directions:

Heat up a pan with the oil, and butter over medium heat, add the garlic, bell pepper, and pepper flakes, stir, and cook for 1 minute. Add the zucchini noodles, stir, and cook for 2 minutes. Add the basil, Parmesan cheese, salt, and pepper, stir, and cook for a few seconds more. Take off the heat, transfer to a bowl, and serve with Asiago cheese on top.

Nutrition: Calories - 140, Fat - 3, Fiber - 1, Carbs - 1. 3, Protein - 5

Bacon and Zucchini Noodles Salad

Preparation time: 10 minutes
Cooking time: 0 minutes
Servings: 2

Ingredients:
- 1 cup baby spinach
- 4 cups zucchini noodles
- ⅓ cup blue cheese, crumbled
- ⅓ cup blue cheese dressing
- ½ cup bacon, cooked and crumbled
- Ground black pepper, to taste

Directions:

In a salad bowl, mix the spinach with the zucchini noodles, bacon, and blue cheese, and toss. Add the cheese dressing and black pepper to the taste, toss well to coat, divide into 2 bowls, and serve.

Nutrition: Calories - 200, Fat - 14, Fiber - 4, Carbs - 2, Protein - 10

Chicken Salad

Preparation time: 10 minutes
Cooking time: 0 minutes
Servings: 3

Ingredients:
- 1 green onion, peeled and chopped
- 1 celery stalk, chopped
- 1 egg, hard-boiled, peeled and chopped
- 5 ounces chicken breast, roasted and chopped
- 2 tablespoons fresh parsley, chopped
- ½ tablespoons dill relish
- Salt and ground black pepper, to taste
- ⅓ cup mayonnaise
- A pinch of garlic powder
- 1 teaspoon mustard

Directions:
In a food processor, mix the parsley with onion, and celery, and pulse well. Transfer these to a bowl, and set aside. Put the chicken in a food processor, blend well, and add to the bowl with the vegetables. Add the egg pieces, salt, and pepper, and stir. Add mustard, mayonnaise, dill relish, and garlic powder, toss to coat, and serve.

Nutrition: Calories - 283, Fat - 23, Fiber - 5, Carbs - 3, Protein - 12

Steak Salad

Preparation time: 10 minutes
Cooking time: 20 minutes
Servings: 4

Ingredients:
- 1½ pound steak, sliced thin
- 3 tablespoons avocado oil
- Salt and ground black pepper, to taste
- ¼ cup balsamic vinegar
- 6 ounces sweet onion, peeled and chopped
- 1 lettuce head, chopped
- 2 garlic cloves, peeled and minced
- 4 ounces mushrooms, sliced
- 1 avocado, pitted, peeled, and sliced
- 3 ounces sundried tomatoes, cored and chopped
- 1 yellow bell pepper, seeded and sliced
- 1 orange bell pepper, seeded and sliced
- 1 teaspoon Italian seasoning
- 1 teaspoon red pepper flakes
- 1 teaspoon onion powder

Directions:
In a bowl, mix the steak pieces with some salt, pepper, and balsamic vinegar, toss to coat, and set aside. Heat up a pan with the avocado oil over medium-low heat, add the mushrooms, garlic, salt, pepper, and onion, stir, and cook for 20 minutes. In a bowl, mix the lettuce leaves with the bell peppers, sundried tomatoes, and avocado, and stirred. Season the steak pieces with the onion powder, pepper flakes, and Italian seasoning. Place the steak pieces in a broiling pan, place under a preheated broiler, and cook for 5 minutes. Divide the steak pieces on plates, add the lettuce, and avocado salad on the side, and top everything with onion, and mushroom mixture.

Nutrition: Calories - 435, Fat - 23, Fiber - 7, Carbs - 10, Protein - 35

Fennel and Chicken Salad

Preparation time: 10 minutes
Cooking time: 0 minutes
Servings: 4

Ingredients:
- 3 chicken breasts, boneless, skinless, cooked, and chopped
- 2 tablespoons walnut oil
- ¼ cup walnuts, toasted and chopped
- 1½ cup fennel, chopped
- 2 tablespoons lemon juice
- ¼ cup mayonnaise
- 2 tablespoons fennel fronds, chopped
- Salt and ground black pepper, to taste
- A pinch of cayenne pepper

Directions:
In a bowl, mix the fennel with chicken, and walnuts, and stir. In another bowl, mix the mayo with salt, pepper, fennel fronds, walnut oil, lemon juice, cayenne, and garlic, and stir well. Pour this over chicken, and fennel mixture, toss to coat well, and keep in the refrigerator until ready to serve.

Nutrition: Calories - 200, Fat - 10, Fiber - 1, Carbs - 3, Protein – 7

Easy Stuffed Avocado

Preparation time: 10 minutes
Cooking time: 0 minutes
Servings: 1

Ingredients:
- 1 avocado
- 4 ounces canned sardines, drained
- 1 green onion, peeled and chopped
- 1 tablespoon mayonnaise
- 1 tablespoon lemon juice
- Salt and ground black pepper, to taste
- ¼ teaspoon turmeric

Directions:
Cut the avocado in half, scoop out the flesh, and put in a bowl. Mix with the sardines and mash with a fork. Mix with the onion, lemon juice, turmeric, salt, pepper, and mayonnaise. Stir everything, divide into avocado halves, and serve.

Nutrition: Calories - 230, Fat - 34, Fiber - 12, Carbs - 5, Protein - 27

Pesto Chicken Salad

Preparation time: 10 minutes
Cooking time: 0 minutes
Servings: 4

Ingredients:
- 1 pound chicken meat, cooked, and cubed
- Salt and ground black pepper, to taste
- 10 cherry tomatoes, halved
- 6 bacon slices, cooked and crumbled
- ¼ cup mayonnaise
- 1 avocado, pitted, peeled, and cubed
- 1 garlic clove, peeled and minced
- 2 tablespoons pesto

Directions:
In a salad bowl, mix the chicken with the bacon, avocado, tomatoes, salt, and pepper, and stir. Add the mayonnaise and garlic pesto, toss well to coat, and serve.

Nutrition: Calories - 357, Fat - 23, Fiber - 5, Carbs - 3, Protein - 26

Chimichurri Steak Salad

Preparation time: 10 minutes
Cooking time: 10 minutes
Servings: 1

Ingredients:
- 4 ounces beef steak
- 2 cups lettuce leaves, shredded
- Salt and ground black pepper, to taste
- Vegetable oil cooking spray
- 2 tablespoons fresh cilantro, chopped
- 2 radishes, sliced
- ⅓ cup red cabbage, shredded
- 3 tablespoons jarred chimichurri sauce
- 1 tablespoons salad dressing
- 3 garlic cloves, peeled and minced
- ½ teaspoon Worcestershire sauce
- 1 tablespoon mustard
- ½ cup apple cider vinegar
- ¼ cup water
- ½ cup olive oil
- ¼ teaspoon hot sauce
- Salt and ground black pepper, to taste

For the salad dressing:

Directions:
In a bowl, mix the garlic cloves with the Worcestershire sauce, mustard, cider vinegar, water, olive oil, salt, pepper, and hot sauce, whisk, and set aside. Heat up a kitchen grill over medium-high heat, spray cooking oil, add the steak, season with salt, and pepper, cook for 4 minutes, flip, cook for 4 minutes, take off the heat, set aside to cool down, and cut into thin strips. In a salad bowl, mix the lettuce with the cilantro, cabbage, radishes, chimichurri sauce, and steak strips. Add the 1 tablespoons of salad dressing, toss to coat, and serve.

Nutrition: Calories - 456, Fat - 32, Fiber - 2, Carbs - 6, Protein - 30

Easy Crab Cakes

- 1 pound crabmeat
- ¼ cup fresh parsley, chopped
- Salt and ground black pepper, to taste
- 2 green onions, chopped
- ¼ cup fresh cilantro, chopped
- 1 teaspoon jalapeño pepper, minced
- 1 teaspoon lemon juice
- 1 teaspoon Worcestershire sauce
- 1 teaspoon Old Bay Seasoning
- ½ teaspoon dry mustard
- ½ cup mayonnaise
- 1 egg
- 2 tablespoons olive oil

Directions:
In a large bowl, mix the crab meat with salt, pepper, parsley, green onions, cilantro, jalapeño, lemon juice, Old Bay seasoning, dry mustard, and Worcestershire sauce, and stir well. In another bowl, mix the egg with the mayonnaise and whisk. Add this to the crabmeat mixture and stir. Shape 6 patties from this mixture, and place them on a plate. Heat up a pan with the oil over medium-high heat, add 3 of the crab cakes, cook for 3 minutes, flip, cook them for 3 minutes, and transfer to paper towels. Repeat with the other 3 crab cakes, drain the excess grease, and serve.

Nutrition: Calories - 254, Fat - 17, Fiber - 1, Carbs - 1, Protein - 20

Lunch Muffins

Preparation time: 10 minutes
Cooking time: 45 minutes
Servings: 13

Ingredients:
- 6 egg yolks
- 2 tablespoons coconut aminos
- ½ pound mushrooms
- ¾ cup coconut flour
- 1 pound ground beef
- Salt, to taste

Directions:
In a food processor, mix the mushrooms with salt, coconut aminos, and egg yolks, and blend well. In a bowl, mix the beef meat with some salt, and stir. Add the mushroom mixture to beef, and stir. Add the coconut flour, and stir again. Divide this into 13 cupcake cups, place in an oven at 350ºF, and bake for 45 minutes. Serve warm.

Nutrition: Calories - 160, Fat - 10, Fiber - 3, Carbs - 1, Protein - 12

Pork Pie

Preparation time: 10 minutes
Cooking time: 50 minutes
Servings: 6

Ingredients:
For the pie crust:
- 2 cups pork cracklings
- ¼ cup flax meal
- 1 cup almond flour
- 2 eggs
- A pinch of salt

For the filling:
- 1 cup cheddar cheese, grated
- 4 eggs
- 12 ounces pork loin, chopped
- 6 bacon slices
- ½ cup cream cheese
- 1 onion, peeled and chopped
- ¼ cup fresh chives, chopped
- 2 garlic cloves, peeled and minced
- Salt and ground black pepper, to taste
- 2 tablespoons butter

Directions:
In a food processor, mix the cracklings with almond flour, flax meal, 2 eggs, and salt, and blend until you obtain a dough. Transfer this to a pie pan, and press on the bottom firmly. Place in an oven at 350°F, and bake for 15 minutes. Heat up a pan with the butter over medium-high heat, add the garlic and onion, stir, and cook for 5 minutes. Add the bacon, stir, and cook for 5 minutes. Add the pork loin, cook until brown on all sides, and take off the heat. In a bowl, mix the eggs with salt, pepper, cheddar cheese, and cream cheese, and blend well. Add the chives, and stir again. Spread pork into pie pan, add the eggs mixture, place in an oven at 350°F, and bake for 25 minutes. Let the pie cool down for a couple of minutes and serve.

Nutrition: Calories - 455, Fat - 34, Fiber - 3, Carbs - 3, Protein - 33

Lunch Pâte

Preparation time: 10 minutes
Cooking time: 0 minutes
Servings: 1

Ingredients:
- 4 ounces chicken livers, sautéed
- ½ teaspoon fresh thyme, chopped
- ½ teaspoon fresh sage, chopped
- ½ teaspoon fresh oregano, chopped
- Salt and ground black pepper, to taste
- 3 tablespoons butter
- 3 radishes, sliced thin
- Crusted bread slices, for serving

Directions:
In a food processor, mix the chicken livers with the thyme, sage, oregano, butter, salt, and pepper, and blend well for a few minutes. Spread on crusted bread slices, and top with radishes slices.

Nutrition: Calories - 380, Fat - 40, Fiber - 5, Carbs - 1, Protein - 17

Chicken Chowder

Preparation time: 10 minutes
Cooking time: 4 hours
Servings: 4

Ingredients:
- 1 pound chicken thighs, skinless and boneless
- 10 ounces canned diced tomatoes
- 1 cup chicken stock
- 8 ounces cream cheese
- Juice from 1 lime
- Salt and ground black pepper, to taste
- 1 jalapeño pepper, chopped
- 1 onion, peeled and chopped
- 2 tablespoons fresh cilantro, chopped
- 1 garlic clove, peeled and minced
- Cheddar cheese, shredded, for serving
- Lime wedges, for serving

Directions:
In a slow cooker, mix the chicken with the tomatoes, stock, cream cheese, salt, pepper, lime juice, jalapeño, onion, garlic, and cilantro, stir, cover, and cook on high for 4 hours. Uncover the slow cooker, shred the meat, divide into bowls, and serve with cheddar cheese on top and lime wedges on the side.

Nutrition: Calories - 300, Fat - 5, Fiber - 6, Carbs - 3, Protein - 26

Coconut Soup

Preparation time: 10 minutes
Cooking time: 30 minutes
Servings: 2

Ingredients:
- 4 cups chicken stock
- 3 lime leaves
- 1½ cups coconut milk
- 1 teaspoon fried lemongrass
- 1 cup fresh cilantro, chopped
- 1-inch fresh ginger, peeled and grated
- 4 Thai chilies, dried and chopped
- Salt and ground black pepper, to taste
- 4 ounces shrimp, peeled and deveined
- 2 tablespoons onion, chopped
- 1 tablespoon coconut oil
- 2 tablespoons mushrooms, chopped
- 1 tablespoon fish sauce
- 1 tablespoon fresh cilantro, chopped
- Juice from 1 lime

Directions:
In a pot, mix the chicken stock with coconut milk, lime leaves, lemongrass, Thai chilies, 1 cup cilantro, ginger, salt, and pepper, stir, bring to a simmer over medium heat, cook for 20 minutes, strain, and return to pot. Heat up the soup again over medium heat, add the coconut oil, shrimp, fish sauce, mushrooms, and onions, stir, and cook for 10 minutes. Add the lime juice, and 1 tablespoon cilantro, stir, ladle into bowls, and serve.

Nutrition: Calories - 450, Fat - 34, Fiber - 4, Carbs - 8, Protein - 12

Zucchini Noodles Soup

Preparation time: 10 minutes
Cooking time: 15 minutes
Servings: 8

Ingredients:

- 1 onion, peeled and chopped
- 2 garlic cloves, peeled and minced
- 1 jalapeño pepper, chopped
- 1 tablespoon coconut oil
- 1½ tablespoons curry paste
- 6 cups chicken stock
- 15 ounces canned coconut milk
- 1 pound chicken breasts, boneless, skinless, and sliced
- 1 red bell pepper, seeded and sliced
- 2 tablespoons fish sauce
- 2 zucchini, cut with a spiralizer
- ½ cup fresh cilantro, chopped
- Lime wedges, for serving

Directions:
Heat up a pot with the oil over medium heat, add the onion, stir, and cook for 5 minutes. Add the garlic, jalapeño, and curry paste, stir, and cook for 1 minute. Add the stock, and coconut milk, stir, and bring to a boil. Add the red bell pepper, chicken, and fish sauce, stir, and simmer for 4 minutes. Add the cilantro, stir, cook for 1 minute, and take off the heat. Divide the zucchini noodles into soup bowls, add the soup on top, and serve with lime wedges on the side.

Nutrition: Calories - 287, Fat - 14, Fiber - 2, Carbs - 7, Protein - 25

Lunch Curry

Preparation time: 10 minutes
Cooking time: 1 hour
Servings: 4

Ingredients:

- 3 tomatoes, cored and chopped
- 2 tablespoons olive oil
- 1 cup chicken stock
- 14 ounces canned coconut milk
- 1 tablespoon lime juice
- Salt and ground black pepper, to taste
- 2 pounds chicken thighs, boneless, skinless, and cubed
- 2 garlic cloves, peeled and minced
- 1 cup onion, peeled and chopped
- 3 red chilies, chopped
- 1 ounce peanuts, toasted
- 1 tablespoon water
- 1 tablespoon fresh ginger, grated
- 2 teaspoons coriander
- 1 teaspoon ground cinnamon
- 1 teaspoon turmeric
- 1 teaspoon cumin
- ½ teaspoon ground black pepper
- 1 teaspoon ground fennel seeds

Directions:
In a food processor, mix the onion with the garlic, peanuts, red chilies, water, ginger, coriander, cinnamon, turmeric, cumin, fennel, and black pepper, blend until you obtain a paste, and set aside. Heat up a pan with the olive oil over medium-high heat, add the spice paste you've made, stir well, and heat up for a few seconds. Add the chicken pieces, stir, and cook for 2 minutes. Add the stock, and tomatoes, stir, reduce heat to low, and cook for 30 minutes. Add the coconut milk, stir, and cook for 20 minutes. Add the salt, pepper, and lime juice, stir, divide into bowls, and serve.

Nutrition: Calories - 430, Fat - 22, Fiber - 4, Carbs - 7, Protein - 53

Spinach Rolls

Preparation time: 20 minutes
Cooking time: 15 minutes
Servings: 16

Ingredients:
- 6 tablespoons coconut flour
- ½ cup almond flour
- 2, and ½ cups mozzarella cheese, shredded
- 2 eggs
- A pinch of salt

For the filling:
- 4 ounces cream cheese
- 6 ounces spinach, torn
- A drizzle of avocado oil
- A pinch of salt
- ¼ cup Parmesan cheese, grated
- Mayonnaise, for serving

Directions:
Heat up a pan with the oil over medium heat, add the spinach, and cook for 2 minutes. Add the Parmesan cheese, a pinch of salt, and cream cheese, stir well, take off the heat, and set aside. Put the mozzarella cheese in a heatproof bowl and microwave for 30 seconds. Add the eggs, salt, coconut, and almond flour, and stir. Place the dough on a lined cutting board, place a parchment paper on top, and flatten dough with a rolling pin. Divide the dough into 16 rectangles, spread spinach mixture on each, and roll them into cigar shapes. Place all rolls on a lined baking sheet, place in an oven at 350ºF, and bake for 15 minutes. Let the rolls cool down for a few minutes before serving them with some mayonnaise on top.

Nutrition: Calories - 500, Fat - 65, Fiber - 4, Carbs - 14, Protein - 32

Steak Bowl

Preparation time: 15 minutes
Cooking time: 8 minutes
Servings: 4

Ingredients:
- 16 ounces skirt steak
- 4 ounces pepper jack cheese, shredded
- 1 cup sour cream
- Salt and ground black pepper, to taste
- ½ cup fresh cilantro, chopped
- A splash of chipotle adobo sauce

For the guacamole:
- ¼ cup onion, chopped
- 2 avocados, pitted and peeled
- Juice from 1 lime
- 1 tablespoon olive oil
- 6 cherry tomatoes, cored and chopped
- 1 garlic clove, peeled and minced
- 1 tablespoon fresh cilantro, chopped
- Salt and ground black pepper, to taste

Directions:
Put the avocados in a bowl and mash with a fork. Add the tomatoes, onion, garlic, salt, and pepper, and stir well. Add the olive oil, lime juice, and 1 tablespoon cilantro, stir again well, and set aside. Heat up a pan over high heat, add the steak, season with salt, and pepper, cook for 4 minutes on each side, transfer to a cutting board, set aside to cool, and cut into thin strips. Divide the steak into 4 bowls, add the cheese, sour cream, and guacamole on top, and serve with a splash of chipotle adobo sauce.

Nutrition: Calories - 600, Fat - 50, Fiber - 6, Carbs - 5, Protein - 30

Meatball Pilaf

Preparation time: 10 minutes
Cooking time: 30 minutes
Servings: 4

Ingredients:
- 12 ounces cauliflower florets
- Salt and ground black pepper, to taste
- 1 egg
- 1 pound ground lamb
- 1 teaspoon fennel seed
- 1 teaspoon paprika
- 1 teaspoon garlic powder
- 1 onion, peeled and chopped
- 2 garlic cloves, peeled and minced
- 2 tablespoons coconut oil
- 1 bunch fresh mint, chopped
- 1 tablespoon lemon zest
- 4 ounces goat cheese, crumbled

Directions:
Put the cauliflower florets in a food processor, add the salt, and pulse well. Grease a pan with some of the coconut oil, heat up over medium heat, add the cauliflower rice, cook for 8 minutes, season with some salt and pepper, take off the heat, and keep warm. In a bowl, mix the lamb with salt, pepper, egg, paprika, garlic powder, and fennel seed, and stir well. Shape 12 meatballs, and place them on a plate for now. Heat up a pan with the coconut oil over medium heat, add the onion, stir, and cook for 6 minutes. Add the garlic, stir, and cook for 1 minute. Add the meatballs, cook them well on all sides, and take off the heat. Divide the cauliflower rice on plates, add the meatballs, and onion mixture on top, sprinkle the mint, lemon zest, and goat cheese at the end, and serve.

Nutrition: Calories - 470, Fat - 43, Fiber - 5, Carbs - 4, Protein - 26

Broccoli Soup

Preparation time: 10 minutes
Cooking time: 30 minutes
Servings: 4

Ingredients:
- 1 white onion, peeled and chopped
- 1 tablespoon butter
- 2 cups vegetable stock
- Salt and ground black pepper, to taste
- 2 cups water
- 2 garlic cloves, peeled and minced
- 1 cup heavy cream
- 8 ounces cheddar cheese, grated
- 12 ounces broccoli florets
- ½ teaspoon paprika

Directions:
Heat up a pot with the butter over medium heat, add the onion and garlic, stir, and cook for 5 minutes. Add the stock, cream, water, salt, pepper, and paprika, stir, and bring to a boil. Add the broccoli, stir, and simmer the soup for 25 minutes. Transfer to a food processor and blend well. Add the cheese and blend again. Divide into soup bowls and serve hot.

Nutrition: Calories - 350, Fat - 34, Fiber - 7, Carbs - 7, Protein - 11

Green Beans Salad

Preparation time: 10 minutes
Cooking time: 5 minutes
Servings: 8

Ingredients:
- 2 tablespoons white wine vinegar
- 1½ tablespoons mustard
- Salt and ground black pepper, to taste
- 2 pounds green beans
- ⅓ cup extra virgin olive oil
- 1½ cups fennel, sliced thin
- 4 ounces goat cheese, crumbled
- ¾ cup walnuts, toasted and chopped

Directions:
Put the water in a pot, add some salt, and bring to a boil over medium-high heat. Add the green beans, cook for 5 minutes, and transfer them to a bowl filled with ice water. Drain the green beans well and put them in a salad bowl. Add the walnuts, fennel, and goat cheese and toss gently. In a bowl, mix the vinegar with the mustard, salt, pepper, and oil, and whisk. Pour this over the salad, toss to coat well, and serve.

Nutrition: Calories - 200, Fat - 14, Fiber - 4, Carbs - 5, Protein - 6

Pumpkin Soup

Preparation time: 10 minutes
Cooking time: 20 minutes
Servings: 6

Ingredients:
- ½ cup onion, peeled and chopped
- 2 tablespoons olive oil
- 1 tablespoon chipotles in adobo sauce
- 1 garlic clove, peeled and minced
- 1 teaspoon cumin
- 1 teaspoon coriander
- A pinch of allspice
- 2 cups pumpkin puree
- Salt and ground black pepper, to taste
- 1 quart chicken stock
- ½ cup heavy cream
- 2 teaspoons vinegar
- 2 teaspoons stevia

Directions:
Heat up a pot with the oil over medium heat, add the onions and garlic, stir, and cook for 4 minutes. Add the stevia, coriander, chipotles, and cumin, stir, and cook for 2 minutes. Add the stock and pumpkin puree, stir, and cook for 5 minutes. Blend the soup well using an immersion blender and then mix with salt, pepper, heavy cream, and vinegar. Stir, cook for 5 minutes, and divide into bowls, and serve.

Nutrition: Calories - 140, Fat - 12, Fiber - 3, Carbs - 6, Protein - 2

Green Bean Casserole

Preparation time: 10 minutes
Cooking time: 35 minutes
Servings: 8

Ingredients:
- 1 pound green beans, halved
- Salt and ground black pepper, to taste
- ½ cup almond flour
- 2 tablespoons butter
- 8 ounces mushrooms, chopped
- 4 ounces onion, peeled and chopped
- 2 shallots, peeled and chopped
- 3 garlic cloves, peeled and minced
- ½ cup chicken stock
- ½ cup heavy cream
- ¼ cup Parmesan cheese, grated
- Avocado oil for frying

Directions:
Put some water in a pot, add the salt, bring to a boil over medium-high heat, add the green beans, cook for 5 minutes, transfer to a bowl filled with ice water, cool down, drain well, and set aside. In a bowl, mix the shallots with the onions, almond flour, salt, and pepper, and toss to coat. Heat up a pan with some avocado oil over medium-high heat, add the onions, and shallots mixture, fry until golden. Transfer to paper towels, and drain the grease. Heat up the pan over medium heat, add the butter, and melt it. Add the garlic and mushrooms, stir, and cook for 5 minutes. Add the stock and heavy cream, stir, bring to a boil, and simmer until it thickens. Add the Parmesan cheese and green beans, toss to coat, and take off the heat. Transfer this mixture to a baking dish, sprinkle some crispy onions mixture all over, place in an oven at 400°F, and bake for 15 minutes. Serve warm.

Nutrition: Calories - 155, fat, 11, Fiber - 6, Carbs - 8, Protein - 5

Apple Salad

Preparation time: 10 minutes
Cooking time: 0 minutes
Servings: 4

Ingredients:

- 2 cups broccoli florets, chopped
- 2 ounces pecans, chopped
- 1 apple, cored and grated
- 1 green onion, diced
- Salt and ground black pepper, to taste
- 2 teaspoons poppy seeds
- 1 teaspoon apple cider vinegar
- ¼ cup mayonnaise
- ½ teaspoon lemon juice
- ¼ cup sour cream

Directions:
In a salad bowl, mix the apple with the broccoli, green onion, and pecans, and stir. Add the poppy seeds, salt, and pepper, and toss gently. In a bowl, mix the mayonnaise with sour cream, vinegar, and lemon juice, and whisk. Pour this over the salad, toss to coat well, and serve cold for lunch.

Nutrition: Calories - 250, Fat - 23, Fiber - 4, Carbs - 4, Protein - 5

Brussels Sprout Gratin

Preparation time: 10 minutes
Cooking time: 35 minutes
Servings: 4

Ingredients:

- 2 ounces onions, diced
- 1 teaspoon garlic, minced
- 6 ounces Brussels sprouts, chopped
- 2 tablespoons butter
- 1 tablespoon coconut aminos
- Salt and ground black pepper, to taste
- ½ teaspoon liquid smoke

For the sauce:
- 2. 5 ounces cheddar cheese, grated
- A pinch of black pepper
- 1 tablespoon butter
- ½ cup heavy cream
- ¼ teaspoon turmeric
- ¼ teaspoon paprika
- A pinch of xanthan gum

For the pork crust:
- 3 tablespoons Parmesan cheese
- ½ ounces pork rinds
- ½ teaspoon sweet paprika

Directions:
Heat up a pan with 2 tablespoons butter over high heat, add the Brussels sprouts, salt, and pepper, stir, and cook for 3 minutes. Add the garlic and onion, stir, and cook for 3 minutes. Add the liquid smoke and coconut aminos, stir, take off the heat, and set aside. Heat up another pan with 1 tablespoon butter over medium heat, add the heavy cream, and stir. Add the cheese, black pepper, turmeric, paprika, and xanthan gum, stir, and cook until it thickens again. Add the Brussels sprouts mixture, toss to coat, and divide into ramekins. In a food processor, mix the Parmesan cheese with the pork rinds, and ½ teaspoon paprika, and pulse well. Divide these crumbs on top of Brussels sprouts mixture, introduce ramekins in the oven at 375°F, and bake for 20 minutes, and serve.

Nutrition: Calories - 300, Fat - 20, Fiber - 6, Carbs - 5, Protein - 10

Fried Asparagus

Preparation time: 10 minutes
Cooking time: 10 minutes
Servings: 4

Ingredients:

- 2 egg yolks
- Salt and ground black pepper, to taste
- ¼ cup butter
- 1 tablespoon lemon juice
- A pinch of cayenne pepper
- 40 asparagus spears

Directions:
In a bowl, whisk the egg yolks well. Transfer this to a small pan over low heat. Add the lemon juice, and whisk. Add the butter and whisk until it melts. Add the salt, pepper, and cayenne pepper, and whisk again. Heat up a pan over medium-high heat, add the asparagus spears, and fry them for 5 minutes. Divide the asparagus on plates, drizzle with the sauce on top, and serve.

Nutrition: Calories - 150, Fat - 13, Fiber - 6, Carbs - 2, Protein - 3

Shrimp Pasta

Preparation time: 10 minutes
Cooking time: 10 minutes
Servings: 4

Ingredients:
- 12 ounces angel hair pasta
- 2 tablespoons olive oil
- Salt and ground black pepper, to taste
- 2 tablespoons butter
- 4 garlic cloves, peeled and minced
- 1 pound shrimp, peeled and deveined
- Juice of ½ lemon
- ½ teaspoon paprika
- ½ cup fresh basil, chopped

Directions:
Put water in a pot, add the some salt, bring to a boil, add the pasta, cook for 2 minutes, drain them, and transfer to a heated pan. Toast the noodles for a few seconds, take off the heat, and leave them aside. Heat up a pan with the butter, and olive oil over medium heat, add the garlic, stir, and brown for 1 minute. Add the shrimp, and lemon juice, and cook for 3 minutes on each side. Add the noodles, salt, pepper, and paprika, stir, divide into bowls, and serve with chopped basil on top.

Nutrition: Calories - 300, Fat - 20, Fiber - 6, Carbs - 3, Protein - 30

Mexican Casserole

Preparation time: 10 minutes
Cooking time: 35 minutes
Servings: 6

Ingredients:
- 2 chipotle peppers, chopped
- 2 jalapeños, chopped
- 1 tablespoon olive oil
- ¼ cup heavy cream
- 1 small white onion, peeled and chopped
- Salt and ground black pepper, to taste
- 1 pound chicken thighs, skinless, boneless, and chopped
- 1 cup red enchilada sauce
- 4 ounces cream cheese
- Vegetable oil cooking spray
- 1 cup pepper jack cheese, shredded
- 2 tablespoons fresh cilantro, chopped
- 2 tortillas

Directions:
Heat up a pan with the oil over medium heat, add the chipotle peppers and jalapeño peppers, stir, and cook for a few seconds. Add the onion, stir, and cook for 5 minutes. Add the cream cheese and heavy cream, and stir until cheese melts. Add the chicken, salt, pepper, and enchilada sauce, stir well, and take off the heat. Grease a baking dish with cooking spray, place the tortillas on the bottom, spread the chicken mixture all over, and sprinkle with shredded cheese. Cover with aluminum foil, place in an oven at 350°F, and bake for 15 minutes. Remove the aluminum foil, and bake for 15 minutes. Sprinkle cilantro on top and serve.

Nutrition: Calories - 240, Fat - 12, Fiber - 5, Carbs - 5, Protein - 20

Asian Salad

Preparation time: 10 minutes
Cooking time: 15 minutes
Servings: 4

Ingredients:
- 1 pound ground beef
- 1 tablespoon sriracha
- 2 tablespoons coconut aminos
- 2 garlic cloves, peeled and minced
- 10 ounces coleslaw mix
- 2 tablespoon sesame seed oil
- Salt and ground black pepper, to taste
- 1 teaspoon apple cider vinegar
- 1 teaspoon sesame seeds
- 1 green onion, chopped

Directions:
Heat up a pan with the oil over medium heat, add the garlic, and brown for 1 minute. Add the beef, stir, and cook for 10 minutes. Add the slaw mixture, toss to coat, and cook for 1minute. Add the vinegar, sriracha, coconut aminos, salt, and pepper, stir, and cook for 4 minutes. Add the green onions and sesame seeds, toss to coat, divide into bowls, and serve.

Nutrition: Calories - 350, Fat - 23, Fiber - 6, Carbs - 3, Protein - 20

Simple Buffalo Wings

Preparation time: 10 minutes
Cooking time: 20 minutes
Servings: 2

Ingredients:
- 2 tablespoons butter
- 6 chicken wings, cut in half
- Salt and ground black pepper, to taste
- A pinch of garlic powder
- ½ cup hot sauce
- A pinch of cayenne pepper
- ½ teaspoon sweet paprika

Directions:
In a bowl, mix the chicken pieces with half of the hot sauce, salt, and pepper, and toss well to coat. Arrange the chicken pieces on a lined baking dish, place under a preheated broiler, and broil 8 minutes. Flip the chicken pieces, and broil for 8 minutes. Heat up a pan with the butter over medium heat. Add the rest of the hot sauce, salt, pepper, cayenne, and paprika, stir, and cook for a couple of minutes. Transfer the broiled chicken pieces to a bowl, add the butter, and hot sauce mixture over them, toss to coat well, and serve.

Nutrition: Calories - 500, Fat - 45, Fiber - 12, Carbs - 1, Protein - 45

Bacon and Mushrooms Skewers

Preparation time: 10 minutes
Cooking time: 20 minutes
Servings: 6

Ingredients:
- 1 pound mushroom caps
- 6 bacon strips
- Salt and ground black pepper, to taste
- ½ teaspoon sweet paprika
- Sweet mesquite seasoning

Directions:
Season the mushroom caps with salt, pepper, and paprika. Spear a bacon strip on a skewer's ends. Spear a mushroom cap, and fold the bacon over it. Repeat until you obtain a mushroom and bacon braid. Repeat with the rest of the mushrooms and bacon strips. Season with sweet mesquite, place all skewers on a preheated kitchen grill over medium heat, cook for 10 minutes, flip, and cook for 10 minutes. Divide on plates and serve.

Nutrition: Calories - 110, Fat - 7, Fiber - 4, Carbs - 2, Protein - 10

Simple Tomato Soup

Preparation time: 10 minutes
Cooking time: 5 minutes
Servings: 4

Ingredients:
- 1 quart canned tomato soup
- 4 tablespoons butter
- ¼ cup olive oil
- ¼ cup red hot sauce
- 2 tablespoons apple cider vinegar
- Salt and ground black pepper, to taste
- 1 teaspoon dried oregano
- 2 teaspoon turmeric
- 8 bacon strips, cooked and crumbled
- ½ cup green onions, chopped
- ½ cup fresh basil leaves, chopped

Directions:
Put the tomato soup in a pot and heat up over medium heat. Add the olive oil, butter, hot sauce, vinegar, salt, pepper, turmeric, and oregano, stir, and simmer for 5 minutes. Take off heat, divide soup into bowls, top with crumbled bacon, basil, and green onions.

Nutrition: Calories - 400, Fat - 34, Fiber - 7, Carbs - 10, Protein - 12

Bacon-wrapped Sausages

Preparation time: 10 minutes
Cooking time: 30 minutes
Servings: 4

Ingredients:
- 8 bacon strips
- 8 sausages
- 16 pepper jack cheese slices
- Salt and ground black pepper, to taste
- A pinch of garlic powder
- ½ teaspoon sweet paprika
- 1 pinch of onion powder

Directions:
Heat up a kitchen grill over medium heat, add the sausages, cook for a few minutes on each side, transfer to a plate, and set aside for a few minutes to cool down. Cut a slit in the middle of each sausage to create pockets, stuff each with 2 cheese slices, and season with salt, pepper, paprika, onion, and garlic powder. Wrap each stuffed sausage in a bacon strip, secure with toothpicks, place on a lined baking sheet, place in an oven at 400ºF, bake for 15 minutes, and serve.

Nutrition: Calories - 500, Fat - 37, Fiber - 12, Carbs - 4, Protein - 40

Lobster Bisque

Preparation time: 10 minutes
Cooking time: 1 hour
Servings: 4

Ingredients:
- 4 garlic cloves, peeled and minced
- 1 onion, peeled and chopped
- 24 ounces lobster chunks, precooked
- Salt and ground black pepper, to taste
- ½ cup tomato paste
- 2 carrots, diced
- 4 celery stalks, chopped
- 1-quart seafood stock
- 1 tablespoon olive oil
- 1 cup heavy cream
- 3 bay leaves
- 1 teaspoon dried thyme
- 1 teaspoon peppercorns
- 1 teaspoon paprika
- 1 teaspoon xanthan gum
- ½ cup fresh parsley, chopped
- 1 tablespoon lemon juice

Directions:
Heat up a pot with the oil over medium heat, add the onion, stir, and cook for 4 minutes. Add the garlic, stir, and cook for 1 minute. Add the celery and carrot, stir, and cook for 1 minute. Add the tomato paste, and stock, and stir. Add the bay leaves, salt, pepper, peppercorns, paprika, thyme, and xanthan gum, stir, and simmer over medium heat for 1 hour. Discard bay leaves, add the cream, and bring to a simmer. Blend using an immersion blender, add the lobster chunks, and cook for a few minutes. Add the lemon juice, stir, divide into bowls, and sprinkle parsley on top.

Nutrition: Calories - 200, Fat - 12, Fiber - 7, Carbs - 6, Protein - 12

Halloumi Salad

Preparation time: 10 minutes
Cooking time: 10 minutes
Servings: 1

Ingredients:
- 3 ounces halloumi cheese, sliced
- 1 cucumber, sliced
- 1 ounce walnuts, chopped
- A drizzle of olive oil
- ½ cup baby arugula
- 5 cherry tomatoes, halved
- A splash of balsamic vinegar
- Salt and ground black pepper, to taste

Directions:
Heat up a kitchen grill over medium-high heat, add the halloumi pieces, grill them for 5 minutes on each side, and transfer to a plate. In a bowl, mix the tomatoes with cucumber, walnuts, and arugula. Add the halloumi pieces on top, season everything with salt, pepper, drizzle the oil, and the vinegar, toss to coat, and serve.

Nutrition: Calories - 450, Fat - 43, Fiber - 5, Carbs - 4, Protein - 21

Beef Shank Stew

Preparation time: 10 minutes
Cooking time: 3 hours and 30 minutes
Servings: 6

Ingredients:

- 8 tomatoes, cored and chopped
- 5 pounds beef shanks
- 3 carrots, peeled and chopped
- 8 garlic cloves, peeled and minced
- 2 onions, peeled and chopped
- 2 cups water
- 1-quart chicken stock
- ¼ cup tomato sauce
- Salt and ground black pepper, to taste
- 2 tablespoons apple cider vinegar
- 3 bay leaves
- 3 teaspoons red pepper, crushed
- 2 teaspoons dried parsley
- 2 teaspoons dried basil
- 2 teaspoons garlic powder
- 2 teaspoons onion powder
- A pinch of cayenne pepper

Directions:
Heat up a pot over medium heat, add the garlic, carrots, and onions, stir, and brown for a few minutes. Heat up a pan over medium heat, add the beef shank, brown for a few minutes on each side, and take off the heat. Add the stock over carrots, the water, and the vinegar, and stir. Add the tomatoes, tomato sauce, salt, pepper, cayenne pepper, crushed pepper, bay leaves, basil, parsley, onion powder, and garlic powder, and stir. Add the beef shanks, cover pot, bring to a simmer, and cook for 3 hours. Discard the bay leaves, divide into bowls, and serve.

Nutrition: Calories - 500, Fat - 22, Fiber - 4, Carbs - 6, Protein - 56

Chicken and Shrimp

Preparation time: 10 minutes
Cooking time: 20 minutes
Servings: 2

Ingredients:

- 20 shrimp, raw, peeled, and deveined
- 2 chicken breasts, boneless, and skinless
- 2 handfuls spinach leaves
- ½ pound mushrooms, chopped
- Salt and ground black pepper, to taste
- ¼ cup mayonnaise
- 2 tablespoons sriracha
- 2 teaspoons lime juice
- 1 tablespoon coconut oil
- ½ teaspoon red pepper, crushed
- 1 teaspoon garlic powder
- ½ teaspoon paprika
- ¼ teaspoon xanthan gum
- 1 green onion, chopped

Directions:
Heat up a pan with the oil over medium-high heat, add the chicken breasts, season with salt, pepper, red pepper, and garlic powder, cook for 8 minutes, flip, and cook for 6 minutes. Add the mushrooms, more salt and pepper, and cook for a few minutes. Heat up another pan over medium heat, add the shrimp, sriracha, paprika, xanthan, and mayonnaise, stir, and cook until shrimp turn pink. Take off heat, add the lime juice, and stir. Divide the spinach on plates, add the chicken and mushroom, top with shrimp mixture, garnish with green onions, and serve.

Nutrition: Calories - 500, Fat - 34, Fiber - 10, Carbs - 3, Protein - 40

Green Soup

Preparation time: 10 minutes
Cooking time: 13 minutes
Servings: 6

Ingredients:
- 1 cauliflower head, separated into florets
- 1 white onion, peeled and diced
- 1 bay leaf, crushed
- 2 garlic cloves, peeled and minced
- 5 ounces watercress
- 7 ounces spinach leaves
- 1 quart vegetable stock
- 1 cup coconut milk
- Salt and ground black pepper, to taste
- ¼ cup butter
- ½ cup parsley, for serving

Directions:
Heat up a pot with the butter over medium-high heat, add the garlic, and onion, stir, and brown for 4 minutes. Add the cauliflower and bay leaf, stir, and cook for 5 minutes. Add the watercress and spinach, stir, and cook for 3 minutes. Add the stock, salt, and pepper, stir, and bring to a boil. Add the coconut milk, stir, take off the heat, and blend using an immersion blender. Divide into bowls and serve.

Nutrition: Calories - 230, Fat - 34, Fiber - 3, Carbs - 5, Protein - 7

Caprese Salad

Preparation time: 5 minutes
Cooking time: 0 minutes
Servings: 2

Ingredients:
- ½ pound mozzarella cheese, sliced
- 1 tomato, sliced
- Salt and ground black pepper, to taste
- 4 basil leaves, torn
- 1 tablespoon balsamic vinegar
- 1 tablespoon olive oil

Directions:
Alternate tomato and mozzarella slices on 2 plates. Sprinkle the salt, pepper, drizzle vinegar, and olive oil. Sprinkle with the basil leaves at the end and serve.

Nutrition: Calories - 150, Fat - 12, Fiber - 5, Carbs - 6, Protein - 9

Salmon Soup

Preparation time: 10 minutes
Cooking time: 25 minutes
Servings: 4

Ingredients:
- 4 leeks, trimmed, and sliced
- Salt and ground black pepper, to taste
- 2 tablespoons avocado oil
- 2 garlic cloves, peeled and minced
- 6 cups chicken stock
- 1 pound salmon, cut into small pieces
- 2 teaspoons dried thyme
- 1¾ cups coconut milk

Directions:
Heat up a pot with the oil over medium heat, add the leeks and garlic, stir, and cook for 5 minutes. Add the thyme, stock, salt, and pepper, stir, and simmer for 15 minutes. Add the coconut milk, and salmon, stir, and bring to a simmer again. Divide into bowls and serve.

Nutrition: Calories - 270, Fat - 12, Fiber - 3, Carbs - 5, Protein - 32

Halibut Soup

Preparation time: 10 minutes
Cooking time: 30 minutes
Servings: 4

Ingredients:
- 1 onion, peeled and chopped
- 1 pound carrots, peeled and sliced
- 1 tablespoon coconut oil
- Salt and ground black pepper, to taste
- 2 tablespoons ginger, minced
- 1 cup water
- 1 pound halibut, cut into medium chunks
- 12 cups chicken stock

Directions:
Heat up a pot with the oil over medium heat, add the onion, stir, and cook for 6 minutes. Add the ginger, carrots, water, and stock, stir bring to a simmer, reduce temperature, and cook for 20 minutes. Blend the soup using an immersion blender, season with salt and pepper, and add the halibut pieces. Stir gently and simmer soup for 5 minutes. Divide into bowls and serve.

Nutrition: Calories - 140, Fat - 6, Fiber - 1, Carbs - 4, Protein - 14

Ketogenic Side Dish Recipes

Simple Kimchi

Preparation time: 1 hour and 10 minutes
Cooking time: 0 minutes
Servings: 6

Ingredients:
- 3 tablespoons salt
- 1 pound napa cabbage, chopped
- 1 carrot, julienned
- ½ cup daikon radish
- 3 green onion stalks, chopped
- 1 tablespoon fish sauce
- 3 tablespoons chili flakes
- 3 garlic cloves, peeled and minced
- 1 tablespoon sesame oil
- ½-inch fresh ginger, peeled and grated

Directions:
In a bowl, mix the cabbage with the salt, massage well for 10 minutes, cover, and set aside for 1 hour. In a bowl, mix the chili flakes with fish sauce, garlic, sesame oil, and ginger, and stir well. Drain the cabbage well, rinse under cold water, and transfer to a bowl. Add the carrots, green onions, radish, and chili paste, and stir. Leave in a dark and cold place for at least 2 days before serving.

Nutrition: Calories - 60, Fat - 3, Fiber - 2, Carbs - 5, Protein - 1

Oven-fried Green Beans

Preparation time: 10 minutes
Cooking time: 10 minutes
Servings: 4

Ingredients:
- ⅔ cup Parmesan cheese, grated
- 1 egg
- 12 ounces green beans
- Salt and ground black pepper, to taste
- ½ teaspoon garlic powder
- ¼ teaspoon paprika

Directions:
In a bowl, mix the Parmesan cheese with salt, pepper, garlic powder, and paprika. In another bowl, whisk the egg with salt and pepper. Dredge the green beans in egg, and then in the Parmesan mixture. Place the green beans on a lined baking sheet, place in an oven at 400°F for 10 minutes. Serve hot.

Nutrition: Calories - 114, Fat - 5, Fiber - 7, Carbs - 3, Protein - 9

Cauliflower Mash

Preparation time: 10 minutes
Cooking time: 10 minutes
Servings: 2

Ingredients:
- ¼ cup sour cream
- 1 small cauliflower head, separated into florets
- Salt and ground black pepper, to taste
- 2 tablespoons feta cheese, crumbled
- 2 tablespoons black olives, pitted and sliced

Directions:
Put water in a pot, add some salt, bring to a boil over medium heat, add the florets, cook for 10 minutes, take off the heat, and drain. Return the cauliflower to the pot, add salt, black pepper, and sour cream, and blend using an immersion blender. Add the black olives and feta cheese, stir, and serve.

Nutrition: Calories - 100, Fat - 4, Fiber - 2, Carbs - 3, Protein - 2

Portobello Mushrooms

Preparation time: 10 minutes
Cooking time: 10 minutes
Servings: 4

Ingredients:
- 12 ounces Portobello mushrooms, sliced
- Salt and ground black pepper, to taste
- ½ teaspoon dried basil
- 2 tablespoons olive oil
- ½ teaspoon tarragon, dried
- ½ teaspoon dried rosemary
- ½ teaspoon dried thyme
- 2 tablespoons balsamic vinegar

Directions:
In a bowl, mix the oil with vinegar, salt, pepper, rosemary, tarragon, basil, and thyme, and whisk. Add the mushroom slices, toss to coat well, place them on a preheated grill over medium-high heat, cook for 5 minutes on both sides, and serve.

Nutrition: Calories - 80, Fat - 4, Fiber - 4, Carbs - 2, Protein - 4

Broiled Brussels Sprouts

Preparation time: 10 minutes
Cooking time: 10 minutes
Servings: 4

Ingredients:
- 1 pound Brussels sprouts, trimmed, and halved
- Salt and ground black pepper, to taste
- 1 teaspoon sesame seeds
- 1 tablespoon green onions, chopped
- 1½ tablespoons sukrin gold syrup
- 1 tablespoon coconut aminos
- 2 tablespoons sesame oil
- 1 tablespoon sriracha

Directions:
In a bowl, mix the sesame oil with coconut aminos, sriracha, syrup, salt, and black pepper, and whisk. Heat up a pan over medium-high heat, add the Brussels sprouts, and cook them for 5 minutes on each side. Add the sesame oil mixture, toss to coat, sprinkle sesame seeds, and green onions, stir again, and serve.

Nutrition: Calories - 110, Fat - 4, Fiber - 4, Carbs - 6, Protein – 4

Pesto

Preparation time: 10 minutes
Cooking time: 0 minutes
Servings: 4

Ingredients:
- ½ cup olive oil
- 2 cups basil
- ⅓ cup pine nuts
- ⅓ cup Parmesan cheese, grated
- 2 garlic cloves, peeled and chopped
- Salt and ground black pepper, to taste

Directions:
Put the basil in a food processor, add the pine nuts, and garlic, and blend well. Add the Parmesan cheese, salt, pepper, and the oil gradually and blend again until you obtain a paste. Serve with chicken or vegetables.

Nutrition: Calories - 100, Fat - 7, Fiber - 3, Carbs - 1, Protein - 5

Brussels Sprouts and Bacon

Preparation time: 10 minutes
Cooking time: 30 minutes
Servings: 4

Ingredients:
- 8 bacon strips, chopped
- 1 pound Brussels sprouts, trimmed, and halved
- Salt and ground black pepper, to taste
- A pinch of cumin
- A pinch of red pepper, crushed
- 2 tablespoons extra virgin olive oil

Directions:
In a bowl, mix the Brussels sprouts with salt, pepper, cumin, red pepper, and oil, and toss to coat. Spread the Brussels sprouts on a lined baking sheet, place in an oven at 375°F, and bake for 30 minutes. Heat up a pan over medium heat, add the bacon pieces, and cook them until they become crispy. Divide the baked Brussels sprouts on plates, top with bacon, and serve.

Nutrition: Calories - 256, Fat - 20, Fiber - 6, Carbs - 5, Protein - 15

Creamy Spinach

Preparation time: 10 minutes
Cooking time: 15 minutes
Servings: 2

Ingredients:
- 2 garlic cloves, peeled and minced
- 8 ounces spinach leaves
- A drizzle of olive oil
- Salt and ground black pepper, to taste
- 4 tablespoons sour cream
- 1 tablespoon butter
- 2 tablespoons Parmesan cheese, grated

Directions:
Heat up a pan with the oil over medium heat, add the spinach, stir and cook until it softens. Add the salt, pepper, butter, Parmesan cheese, and butter, stir, and cook for 4 minutes. Add the sour cream, stir, and cook for 5 minutes. Divide on plates and serve.

Nutrition: Calories - 133, Fat - 10, Fiber - 4, Carbs - 4, Protein - 2

Avocado Fries

Preparation time: 10 minutes
Cooking time: 5 minutes
Servings: 3

Ingredients:
- 3 avocados, pitted, peeled, halved, and sliced
- 1½ cups sunflower oil
- 1½ cups almond meal
- A pinch of cayenne pepper
- Salt and ground black pepper, to taste

Directions:
In a bowl, mix the almond meal with salt, pepper, and cayenne, and stir. In a second bowl, whisk eggs with a pinch of salt, and pepper. Dredge the avocado pieces in egg, and then in almond meal mixture. Heat up a pan with the oil over medium-high heat, add the avocado fries, and cook them until they are golden. Transfer to paper towels, drain grease, and divide on plates and serve.

Nutrition: Calories - 450, Fat - 43, Fiber - 4, Carbs - 7, Protein - 17

Roasted Cauliflower

Preparation time: 10 minutes
Cooking time: 25 minutes
Servings: 6

Ingredients:
- 1 cauliflower head, separated into florets
- Salt and ground black pepper, to taste
- ⅓ cup Parmesan cheese, grated
- 1 tablespoon fresh parsley, chopped
- 3 tablespoons olive oil
- 2 tablespoons extra virgin olive oil

Directions:
In a bowl, mix the oil with garlic, salt, pepper, and cauliflower florets. Toss to coat well, spread this on a lined baking sheet, place in an oven at 450°F, and bake for 25 minutes, stirring halfway. Add the Parmesan cheese, and parsley, stir, and cook for 5 minutes. Divide on plates and serve.

Nutrition: Calories - 118, Fat - 2, Fiber - 3, Carbs - 1, Protein - 6

Mushrooms and Spinach

Preparation time: 10 minutes
Cooking time: 10 minutes
Servings: 4

Ingredients:
- 10 ounces spinach leaves, chopped
- Salt and ground black pepper, to taste
- 14 ounces mushrooms, chopped
- 2 garlic cloves, peeled and minced
- ½ cup fresh parsley, chopped
- 1 onion, peeled and chopped
- 4 tablespoons olive oil
- 2 tablespoons balsamic vinegar

Directions:
Heat up a pan with the oil over medium-high heat, add the garlic and onion, stir, and cook for 4 minutes. Add the mushrooms, stir, and cook for 3 minutes. Add the spinach, stir, and cook for 3 minutes. Add the vinegar, salt, and pepper, stir, and cook for 1 minute. Add the parsley, stir, divide on plates, and serve.

Nutrition: Calories - 200, Fat - 4, Fiber - 6, Carbs - 2, Protein - 12

Okra and Tomatoes

Preparation time: 10 minutes
Cooking time: 10 minutes
Servings: 6

Ingredients:
- 14 ounces canned stewed tomatoes, cored and chopped
- Salt and ground black pepper, to taste
- 2 celery stalks, chopped
- 1 onion, peeled and chopped
- 1 pound okra, trimmed and sliced
- 2 bacon slices, chopped
- 1 small green bell peppers, seeded and chopped

Directions:
Heat up a pan over medium-high heat, add the bacon, stir, brown for a few minutes, transfer to paper towels, and set aside. Heat up the pan again over medium heat, add the okra, bell pepper, onion, and celery, stir, and cook for 2 minutes. Add the tomatoes, salt, and pepper, stir, and cook for 3 minutes. Divide on plates, garnish with crispy bacon, and serve.

Nutrition: Calories - 100, Fat - 2, Fiber - 3, Carbs - 2, Protein - 6

Snap Peas and Mint

Preparation time: 10 minutes
Cooking time: 5 minutes
Servings: 4

Ingredients:
- ¾ pound sugar snap peas, trimmed
- Salt and ground black pepper, to taste
- 1 tablespoon mint leaves, chopped
- 2 teaspoons olive oil
- 3 green onions, chopped
- 1 garlic clove, peeled and minced

Directions:
Heat up a pan with the oil over medium-high heat. Add the snap peas, salt, pepper, green onions, garlic, and mint. Stir everything, cook for 5 minutes, divide on plates, and serve.

Nutrition: Calories - 70, Fat - 1, Fiber - 1, Carbs - 0. 4, Protein - 6

Collard Greens with Turkey

Preparation time: 10 minutes
Cooking time: 2 hours and 15 minutes
Servings: 10

Ingredients:
- 5 bunches collard greens, chopped
- Salt and ground black pepper, to taste
- 1 tablespoon red pepper flakes
- 5 cups chicken stock
- 1 turkey leg
- 2 tablespoons garlic, minced
- ¼ cup olive oil

Directions:
Heat up a pot with the oil over medium heat, add the garlic, stir, and cook for 1 minute. Add the stock, salt, pepper, and turkey leg, stir, cover, and simmer for 30 minutes. Add the collard greens, cover pot again, and cook for 45 minutes. Reduce heat to medium, add more salt and pepper, stir, and cook for 1 hour. Drain the greens, chop up the turkey, mix everything with the red pepper flakes, stir, divide on plates, and serve.

Nutrition: Calories - 143, Fat - 3, Fiber - 4, Carbs - 3, Protein - 6

Eggplant and Tomatoes

Preparation time: 10 minutes
Cooking time: 15 minutes
Servings: 4

Ingredients:
- 1 tomato, sliced
- 1 eggplant, sliced into thin rounds
- Salt and ground black pepper, to taste
- ¼ cup Parmesan cheese, grated
- A drizzle of olive oil

Directions:
Place eggplant slices on a lined baking dish, drizzle some oil, and sprinkle half of the Parmesan. Top eggplant slices with tomato ones, season with some salt and pepper, and sprinkle the rest of the cheese over them.
Place in an oven at 400°F, and bake for 15 minutes. Divide on plates and serve hot as a side dish.

Nutrition: Calories - 55, Fat - 1, Fiber - 1, Carbs - 0. 5, Protein - 7

Broccoli with Lemon Almond Butter

Preparation time: 10 minutes
Cooking time: 10 minutes
Servings: 4

Ingredients:
- 1 broccoli head, separated into florets
- Salt and ground black pepper, to taste
- ¼ cup almonds, blanched
- 1 teaspoon lemon zest
- ¼ cup coconut butter, melted
- 2 tablespoons lemon juice

Directions:
Put water in a pot, add the salt, and bring to a boil over medium-high heat. Place the broccoli florets in a steamer basket, place into the pot, cover, and steam for 8 minutes. Drain and transfer to a bowl. Heat up a pan with the coconut butter over medium heat, add the lemon juice, lemon zest, and almonds, stir, and take off the heat. Add the broccoli, toss to coat, divide on plates, and serve.

Nutrition: Calories - 170, Fat - 15, Fiber - 4, Carbs - 4, Protein - 4

Sautéed Broccoli

Preparation time: 10 minutes
Cooking time: 22 minutes
Servings: 4

Ingredients:
- 5 tablespoons olive oil
- 1 garlic clove, peeled and minced
- 1 pound broccoli florets
- 1 tablespoon Parmesan cheese, grated
- Salt and ground black pepper, to taste

Directions:
Put water in a pot, add the salt, bring to a boil over medium-high heat, add the broccoli, cook for 5 minutes, and drain. Heat up a pan with the oil over medium-high heat, add the garlic, stir, and cook for 2 minutes. Add the broccoli, stir, and cook for 15 minutes. Take off the heat, sprinkle Parmesan cheese, divide on plates, and serve.

Nutrition: Calories - 193, Fat - 14, Fiber - 3, Carbs - 6, Protein - 5

Easy Grilled Onions

Preparation time: 10 minutes
Cooking time: 1 hour
Servings: 4

Ingredients:
- ½ cup butter
- 4 onions
- 4 chicken bouillon cubes
- Salt and ground black pepper, to taste

Direction:
Cut the onion tops make a hole in the middle, divide the butter and chicken bouillon cubes into these holes, and season with salt and pepper. Wrap the onions in aluminum foil, place them on preheated kitchen grill, and grill for 1 hour. Unwrap the onions, chop them into big chunks, arrange on plates, and serve.

Nutrition: Calories - 135, Fat - 11, Fiber - 4, Carbs - 6, Protein - 3

Sautéed Zucchini

Preparation time: 10 minutes
Cooking time: 15 minutes
Servings: 6

Ingredients:
- 1 onion, peeled and chopped
- 1 tomato, cored and chopped
- ½ pound tomatoes, cored and chopped
- Salt and ground black pepper, to taste
- 1 garlic clove, peeled and minced
- 1 teaspoon Italian seasoning
- 4 zucchini, sliced

Directions:
Heat up a pan with the oil over medium heat, add the onion, salt, and pepper, stir, and cook for 2 minutes. Add the mushrooms, and zucchini, stir, and cook for 5 minutes. Add the garlic, tomatoes, and Italian seasoning, stir, cook for 6 minutes. Take off the heat, divide on plates, and serve.

Nutrition: Calories - 70, Fat - 3, Fiber - 2, Carbs - 6, Protein - 4

Fried Swiss Chard

Preparation time: 10 minutes
Cooking time: 10 minutes
Servings: 2

Ingredients:
- 2 tablespoons butter
- 4 bacon slices, chopped
- 1 bunch Swiss chard, chopped
- ½ teaspoon garlic paste
- 3 tablespoons lemon juice
- Salt and ground black pepper, to taste

Directions:
Heat up a pan over medium heat, add the bacon pieces, and cook until it's crispy. Add the butter, and stir until it melts. Add the garlic paste and lemon juice, stir, and cook for 1 minute. Add the Swiss chard, stir, and cook for 4 minutes. Add the salt and black pepper to the taste, stir, divide on plates, and serve.

Nutrition: Calories - 300, Fat - 32, Fiber - 7, Carbs - 6, Protein - 8

Mushroom Salad

Preparation time: 10 minutes
Cooking time: 10 minutes
Servings: 4

Ingredients:
- 2 tablespoons butter
- 1 pound cremini mushrooms, chopped
- 4 tablespoons extra virgin olive oil
- Salt and ground black pepper, to taste
- 4 bunches arugula
- 8 slices prosciutto
- 2 tablespoons apple cider vinegar
- 8 sundried tomatoes in oil, drained, and chopped
- Parmesan cheese, shaved
- Fresh parsley leaves, chopped

Directions:
Heat up a pan with the butter and half of the oil over medium-high heat. Add the mushrooms, salt, and pepper, stir, and cook for 3 minutes. Reduce the heat, stir again, and cook for 3 more minutes. Add the rest of the oil, and the vinegar, stir and cook 1 minute. Place the arugula on a serving platter, add the prosciutto on top, add the mushroom mixture, sundried tomatoes, more salt and pepper, Parmesan shavings, and parsley, and serve.

Nutrition: Calories - 160, Fat - 4, Fiber - 2, Carbs - 2, Protein - 6

Greek Side Salad

Preparation time: 10 minutes
Cooking time: 7 minutes
Servings: 6

Ingredients:
- ½ pounds mushrooms, sliced
- 1 tablespoon extra virgin olive oil
- 3 garlic cloves, peeled and minced
- 1 teaspoon dried basil
- Salt and ground black pepper, to taste
- 1 tomato, cored and diced
- 3 tablespoons lemon juice
- ½ cup water
- 1 tablespoons coriander, chopped

Directions:
Heat up a pan with the oil over medium heat, add the mushrooms, stir, and cook for 3 minutes. Add the basil and garlic, stir, and cook for 1 minute. Add the water, salt, pepper, tomato, and lemon juice, stir, and cook for a few minutes. Take off the heat, transfer to a bowl, set aside to cool down, sprinkle the coriander, and serve.

Nutrition: Calories - 200, Fat - 2, Fiber - 2, Carbs - 1, Protein - 10

Tomato Salsa

Preparation time: 2 hours
Cooking time: 0 minutes
Servings: 5

Ingredients:
- 3 yellow tomatoes, seeded and chopped
- 1 red tomato, seeded and chopped
- Salt and ground black pepper, to taste
- 1 cup watermelon, seeded and chopped
- ⅓ cup onion, diced
- 1 mango, peeled, seeded and chopped
- 2 jalapeño peppers, diced
- ¼ cup cilantro, diced
- 3 tablespoons lime juice
- 2 teaspoons honey

Directions:
In a bowl, mix the tomatoes with mango, watermelon, onion, and jalapeño. Add the cilantro, lime juice, salt, pepper, and honey, and stir well. Cover the bowl, keep in the refrigerator for 2 hours, and serve.

Nutrition: Calories - 80, Fat - 1, Fiber - 2, Carbs - 1, Protein - 4

Summer Side Salad

Preparation time: 10 minutes
Cooking time: 5 minutes
Servings: 6

Ingredients:
- ½ cup extra virgin olive oil
- 1 cucumber, chopped
- 2 baguettes, cut into small cubes
- 2 pints colored cherry tomatoes, cut into half
- Salt and ground black pepper, to taste
- 1 onion, peeled and chopped
- 3 tablespoons balsamic vinegar
- 1 garlic clove, peeled and minced
- 1 bunch fresh basil, chopped

Directions:
In a bowl, mix the bread cubes with half of the oil, and toss to coat. Heat up a pan over medium-high heat, add the bread, stir, toast for 10 minutes, take off the heat, drain, and set aside. In a bowl, mix the vinegar with salt, pepper, and the rest of the oil, and whisk. In a salad bowl, mix the cucumber with tomatoes, onion, garlic, and bread. Add the vinegar dressing, toss to coat, sprinkle the basil, add more salt and pepper, if needed, toss to coat, and serve.

Nutrition: Calories - 90, Fat - 0, Fiber - 2, Carbs - 2, Protein - 4

Tomato and Bocconcini

Preparation time: 6 minutes
Cooking time: 0 minutes
Servings: 4

Ingredients:
- 20 ounces tomatoes, cut in wedges
- 2 tablespoons extra virgin olive oil
- 1½ tablespoons balsamic vinegar
- 1 teaspoon stevia
- 1 garlic clove, minced
- 8 ounces baby bocconcini, drained and torn
- 1 cup fresh basil leaves, chopped
- Salt and ground black pepper, to taste

Directions:
In a bowl, mix the stevia with vinegar, garlic, oil, salt, and pepper, and whisk. In a salad bowl, mix the bocconcini with the tomato and basil. Add the dressing, toss to coat, and serve.

Nutrition: Calories - 100, Fat - 2, Fiber - 2, Carbs - 1, Protein - 9

Cucumber and Date Salad

Preparation time: 10 minutes
Cooking time: 0 minutes
Servings: 4

Ingredients:
- 2 English cucumbers, chopped
- 8 dates, pitted and sliced
- ¾ cup fennel, sliced thin
- 2 tablespoons fresh chives, diced
- ½ cup walnuts, chopped
- 2 tablespoons lemon juice
- 4 tablespoons fruity olive oil
- Salt and ground black pepper, to taste

Directions:
Put the cucumber on a paper towel, press well, and transfer to a salad bowl. Crush them a bit using a fork. Add the dates, fennel, chives, and walnuts, and stir gently. Add the salt, pepper, lemon juice, and the oil, toss to coat, and serve.

Nutrition: Calories - 80, Fat - 0. 2, Fiber - 1, Carbs – 0.4, Protein - 5

Eggplant Salad

Preparation time: 10 minutes
Cooking time: 10 minutes
Servings: 4

Ingredients:
- 1 eggplant, sliced
- 1 onion, peeled and sliced
- A drizzle of canola oil
- 1 avocado, pitted and chopped
- 1 teaspoon mustard
- 1 tablespoon balsamic vinegar
- 1 tablespoon fresh oregano, chopped
- A drizzle of olive oil
- Salt and ground black pepper, to taste
- Zest from 1 lemon
- Fresh parsley, chopped, for serving

Directions:
Brush the onion slices and eggplant ones with a drizzle of canola oil, place them on a heated kitchen grill, and cook them until they become soft. Transfer them to a cutting board, leave them to cool down, chop them, and put them in a bowl. Add the avocado and stir gently. In a bowl, mix the vinegar with mustard, oregano, olive oil, salt and pepper to taste. Add this to the eggplant, avocado, and onion mixture, toss to coat, add the lemon zest and parsley on top, and serve.

Nutrition: Calories - 120, Fat - 3, Fiber - 2, Carbs - 1, Protein - 8

Baked Eggplant Side Salad

Preparation time: 2 hours and 10 minutes
Cooking time: 1 hour and 30 minutes
Servings: 12

Ingredients:
- 1 garlic clove, peeled and crushed
- 6 eggplants
- 1 teaspoon dried parsley
- 1 teaspoon dried oregano
- ¼ teaspoon dried basil
- 3 tablespoons extra virgin olive oil
- 2 tablespoons stevia
- 1 tablespoon balsamic vinegar
- Salt and ground black pepper, to taste

Directions:
Prick the eggplants with a fork, arrange them on a baking sheet, place in an oven at 350ºF, bake for 1 hour and 30 minutes, take them out of the oven, leave them to cool down, peel them, chop them, and transfer them to a salad bowl. Add the garlic, oil, parsley, stevia, oregano, basil, salt, and pepper, toss to coat, keep in the refrigerator for 2 hours, and then serve.

Nutrition: Calories - 150, Fat - 1, Fiber - 2, Carbs - 1, Protein - 8

Endive and Watercress Side Salad

Preparation time: 10 minutes
Cooking time: 5 minutes
Servings: 4

Ingredients:
- 4 medium endives, roots and ends cut and sliced thin crosswise
- 1 tablespoon lemon juice
- 1 shallot, peeled and diced
- 1 tablespoon balsamic vinegar
- 2 tablespoons extra virgin olive oil
- 6 tablespoons heavy cream
- Salt and ground black pepper, to taste
- 4 ounces watercress, chopped
- 1 apple, cored and sliced thin
- 1 tablespoon fresh chervil, chopped
- 1 tablespoon fresh tarragon, chopped
- 1 tablespoon fresh chives, chopped
- ⅓ cup almonds, chopped
- 1 tablespoon fresh parsley, chopped

Directions:
In a bowl, mix the lemon juice with vinegar, salt, and shallot, stir, and set aside for 10 minutes. Add the olive oil, pepper, stir, and set aside for 2 minutes. Put the endives, apple, watercress, chives, tarragon, parsley, and chervil in a salad bowl. Add salt and pepper to taste and toss to coat. Add the heavy cream and vinaigrette, stir gently, and serve with almonds on top.

Nutrition: Calories - 200, Fat - 3, Fiber - 5, Carbs - 2, Protein - 10

Indian Side Salad

Preparation time: 15 minutes
Cooking time: 0 minutes
Servings: 6

Ingredients:
- 3 carrots, peeled and grated
- 2 courgettes, sliced thin
- A bunch of radishes, finely sliced
- ½ onion, peeled and chopped
- 6 mint leaves, chopped

For the salad dressing:
- 1 teaspoon mustard
- 1 tablespoons homemade mayo
- 1 tablespoons balsamic vinegar
- 2 tablespoons extra virgin olive oil
- Salt and ground black pepper, to taste

Directions:
In a bowl, mix the mustard with mayonnaise, vinegar, salt, and pepper, and stir well. Add the oil gradually and whisk everything. In a salad bowl, mix the carrots with radishes, courgettes, and mint leaves. Add the salad dressing, toss to coat, and keep in the refrigerator until ready to serve.

Nutrition: Calories - 140, Fat - 1, Fiber - 2, Carbs - 1, Protein - 7

Indian Mint Chutney

Preparation time: 10 minutes
Cooking time: 0 minutes
Servings: 8

Ingredients:
- 1½ cup mint leaves
- 1 bunch cilantro, stems removed
- Salt and ground black pepper, to taste
- 1 green chili pepper, seedless
- 1 onion, cut into medium-sized chunks
- ¼ cup water
- 1 tablespoon tamarind juice

Directions:
Put the mint and cilantro leaves in a food processor and blend them. Add the chili pepper, salt, black pepper, onion, and tamarind paste and blend again. Add the water, blend some more until you obtain cream, transfer to a bowl, and serve.

Nutrition: Calories - 100, Fat - 1, Fiber - 1, Carbs - 0. 4, Protein - 6

Indian Coconut Chutney

Preparation time: 5 minutes
Cooking time: 5 minutes
Servings: 3

Ingredients:
- ½ teaspoon cumin
- ½ cup coconut, grated
- 2 tablespoons chana dal, already fried
- 2 green chilies
- Salt, to taste
- 1 garlic clove, peeled
- ¾ tablespoons avocado oil
- ¼ teaspoon mustard seeds
- A pinch of hing
- ½ teaspoons urad dal
- 1 red chili chopped
- 1 spring curry leaves

Directions:
In a food processor, mix the coconut with salt, cumin, garlic, chana dal, and green chilies and blend well. Add a splash of water and blend again. Heat up a pan with the oil over medium heat, add the red chili, urad dal, mustard seeds, hing, and curry leaves, stir, and cook for 3 minutes. Add this to coconut chutney, stir gently, and serve.

Nutrition: Calories - 90, Fat - 1, Fiber - 1, Carbs - 1, Protein - 6

Easy Tamarind Chutney

Preparation time: 10 minutes
Cooking time: 35 minutes
Servings: 10

Ingredients:
- 1 teaspoon cumin seeds
- 1 tablespoon canola oil
- ½ teaspoon garam masala
- ½ teaspoon asafetida powder
- 1 teaspoon ground ginger
- ½ teaspoon fennel seeds
- ½ teaspoon cayenne pepper
- 1¼ cups coconut sugar
- 2 cups water
- 3 tablespoons tamarind paste

Directions:
Heat up a pan with the oil over medium heat, add the ginger, cumin, cayenne pepper, asafetida powder, fennel seeds, and garam masala, stir, and cook for 2 minutes. Add the water, sugar, and tamarind paste, stir, bring to a boil, reduce heat to low, and simmer chutney for 30 minutes. Transfer to a bowl, and let it cool down before serving.

Nutrition: Calories - 120, Fat - 1, Fiber - 3, Carbs - 5, Protein - 9

Caramelized Bell Peppers

Preparation time: 10 minutes
Cooking time: 32 minutes
Servings: 4

Ingredients:
- 1 tablespoon olive oil
- 1 teaspoon butter
- 2 red bell peppers, cut into thin strips
- 2 onions, cut into thin strips
- Salt and ground black pepper, to taste
- 1 teaspoon dried basil

Directions:
Heat up a pan with the butter and oil over medium heat, add the onion and bell peppers, stir, and cook for 2 minutes. Reduce the temperature and cook for 30 minutes, stirring often. Add the salt, pepper, and basil, stir again, take off the heat, and serve.

Nutrition: Calories - 97, Fat - 4, Fiber - 2, Carbs - 6, Protein - 2

Caramelized Red Chard

Preparation time: 10 minutes
Cooking time: 20 minutes
Servings: 4

Ingredients:
- 2 tablespoons olive oil
- 1 onion, peeled and chopped
- 2 tablespoons capers
- Juice of 1 lemon
- Salt and ground black pepper, to taste
- 1 teaspoon palm sugar
- 1 bunch red chard, chopped
- ¼ cup Kalamata olives, pitted and chopped

Directions:
Heat up a pan with the oil over medium heat, add the onions, stir, and brown for 4 minutes. Add the palm sugar, and stir well. Add the olives and chard, stir, and cook for 10 minutes. Add the capers, lemon juice, salt, and pepper, stir, and cook for 3 minutes. Divide on plates and serve.

Nutrition: Calories - 119, Fat - 7, Fiber - 3, Carbs - 7, Protein - 2

Summer Kale

Preparation time: 10 minutes
Cooking time: 45 minutes
Servings: 4

Ingredients:
- 2 cups water
- 1 tablespoon balsamic vinegar
- ⅓ cup almonds, toasted
- 3 garlic cloves, peeled and minced
- 1 bunch kale, steamed, and chopped
- 1 onion, peeled and chopped
- 2 tablespoons olive oil

Directions:
Heat up a pan with the oil over medium heat, add the onion, stir, and cook for 10 minutes. Add the garlic, stir, and cook for 1 minute. Add the water and kale, cover the pan, and cook for 30 minutes. Add the salt, pepper, balsamic vinegar, and almonds, toss to coat, divide on plates, and serve.

Nutrition: Calories - 170, Fat - 11, Fiber - 3, Carbs - 7, Protein - 7

Coleslaw

Preparation time: 10 minutes
Cooking time: 0 minutes
Servings: 4

Ingredients:
- 1 small green cabbage head, shredded
- Salt and ground black pepper, to taste
- 6 tablespoons mayonnaise
- Salt and ground black pepper, to taste
- 1 pinch fennel seed
- Juice of ½ lemon
- 1 tablespoon Dijon mustard

Directions:
In a bowl, mix the cabbage with salt and lemon juice, stir well, and set aside for 10 minutes. Add salt, pepper, fennel seed, mayonnaise, and mustard to the cabbage. Toss to coat and serve.

Nutrition: Calories - 150, Fat - 3, Fiber - 2, Carbs - 2, Protein - 7

Fried Cabbage

Preparation time: 10 minutes
Cooking time: 15 minutes
Servings: 4

Ingredients:
- 1½ pound green cabbage, shredded
- Salt and ground black pepper, to taste
- 3. 5 ounces butter
- A pinch of sweet paprika

Directions:
Heat up a pan with the butter over medium heat. Add the cabbage and cook for 15 minutes, stirring often. Add the salt, pepper, and paprika, stir, cook for 1 minute, divide on plates, and serve.

Nutrition: Calories - 200, Fat - 4, Fiber - 2, Carbs - 3, Protein - 7

Green Beans and Avocado

Preparation time: 10 minutes
Cooking time: 5 minutes
Servings: 4

Ingredients:
- ⅔ pound green beans, trimmed
- Salt and ground black pepper, to taste
- 3 tablespoons olive oil
- 2 avocados, pitted and peeled
- 5 scallions, chopped
- ½ cup fresh cilantro, chopped

Directions:
Heat up a pan with the oil over medium heat, add the green beans, stir, and cook for 4 minutes. Add the salt and pepper, stir, take off the heat, and transfer to a bowl. In another bowl, mix the avocados with salt and pepper, and mash with a fork. Add the onions and stir well. Add this over green beans, toss to coat, and serve.

Nutrition: Calories - 200, Fat - 5, Fiber - 3, Carbs - 4, Protein - 6

Creamy Spaghetti Pasta

Preparation time: 10 minutes
Cooking time: 40 minutes
Servings: 4

Ingredients:
- 1 spaghetti squash
- Salt and ground black pepper, to taste
- 2 tablespoons butter
- 1 teaspoon Cajun seasoning
- A pinch of cayenne pepper
- 2 cups heavy cream

Directions:
Prick the squash with a fork, place on a lined baking sheet, place in an oven at 350°F, and bake for 15 minutes. Take the squash out of the oven, set aside to cool, and scoop out the squash flesh. Heat up a pan with the butter over medium heat, add the spaghetti squash, stir, and cook for a couple of minutes. Add salt, pepper, cayenne pepper, and Cajun seasoning, stir, and cook for 1 minute. Add the heavy cream, stir, cook for 10 minutes, divide on plates, and serve.

Nutrition: Calories - 200, Fat - 2, Fiber - 1, Carbs - 5, Protein - 8

Roasted Olives

Preparation time: 10 minutes
Cooking time: 20 minutes
Servings: 6

Ingredients:
- 1 cup black olives, pitted
- 1 cup Kalamata olives, pitted
- 1 cup green olives, stuffed with almonds and garlic
- ¼ cup olive oil
- 10 garlic cloves
- 1 tablespoon herbes de Provence
- 1 teaspoon lemon zest, grated
- Ground black pepper, to taste
- Fresh thyme, chopped, for serving

Directions:
Place black olives, Kalamata olives, and green olives on a lined baking sheet, drizzle oil, garlic, and herbes de Provence, toss to coat, place in an oven at 425°F, and bake for 10 minutes. Stir the olives and bake for 10 minutes. Divide the olives on plates, sprinkle lemon zest, black pepper, and thyme on top, toss to coat, and serve warm.

Nutrition: Calories - 200, Fat - 20, Fiber - 4, Carbs - 3, Protein - 1

Vegetable Noodles

Preparation time: 10 minutes
Cooking time: 20 minutes
Servings: 6

Ingredients:
- 1 zucchini, cut with a spiralizer
- 1 summer squash, cut with a spiralizer
- 1 carrot, cut with a spiralizer
- 1 sweet potato, cut with a spiralizer
- 4 ounces onion, chopped
- 6 ounces yellow, orange, and red bell peppers, seeded and cut into thin strips
- Salt and ground black pepper, to taste
- 4 tablespoons bacon fat
- 3 garlic cloves, peeled and minced

Directions:
Spread the zucchini noodles on a lined baking sheet. Add the squash, carrot, sweet potato, onion, and bell peppers. Add salt, pepper, and garlic and toss to coat. Add the bacon fat, toss again, place in an oven at 400°F, and bake for 20 minutes. Transfer to plates and serve.

Nutrition: Calories - 50, Fat - 1, Fiber - 1, Carbs - 6, Protein - 2

Mustard and Garlic Brussels Sprouts

Preparation time: 10 minutes
Cooking time: 40 minutes
Servings: 4

Ingredients:
- 1 pound Brussels sprouts, trimmed, and halved
- Salt and ground black pepper, to taste
- 1 tablespoon coconut aminos
- 1 tablespoon Dijon mustard
- 1 tablespoon garlic cloves, peeled and minced
- 1 tablespoons butter
- 1 garlic clove head, cloves peeled, and separated
- 1 tablespoon caraway seeds

Directions:
Put the Brussels sprouts on a lined baking sheet. Add the minced garlic, whole garlic, butter, mustard, salt, pepper, coconut aminos, and caraway seeds. Toss to coat well, place in an oven at 400ºF, and bake for 40 minutes. Transfer to plates and serve.

Nutrition: Calories - 70, Fat - 4, Fiber - 2, Carbs - 4, Protein - 2. 4

Cheese Sauce

Preparation time: 10 minutes
Cooking time: 12 minutes
Servings: 8

Ingredients:
- 2 tablespoons butter
- ¼ cup cream cheese, softened
- ¼ cup whipping cream
- ¼ cup cheddar cheese, grated
- 2 tablespoons water
- A pinch of salt
- ¼ teaspoon cayenne pepper
- ½ teaspoon sweet paprika
- ½ teaspoon onion powder
- ½ teaspoon garlic powder
- 4 tablespoons fresh parsley, chopped

Directions:
Heat up a pan with the butter over medium heat. Add the whipping cream and stir well. Add the cream cheese, stir, and bring to a simmer. Take off the heat, add the cheddar cheese, stir, return to the heat, and cook for 3-4 minutes. Add the water, a pinch of salt, cayenne pepper, onion powder, garlic powder, paprika, and parsley, stir well, take off the heat, and serve.

Nutrition: Calories - 200, Fat - 13, Fiber - 0, Carbs - 1, Protein - 6

Sautéed Kohlrabi

Preparation time: 10 minutes
Cooking time: 10 minutes
Servings: 4

Ingredients:
- 2 kohlrabi, trimmed and sliced thin
- Salt and ground black pepper, to taste
- 1 tablespoons fresh parsley, chopped
- 1 tablespoon butter
- 2 garlic cloves, peeled and minced

Directions:
Put some water in a pot and bring to a boil over medium heat. Add the kohlrabi slices, cook for 5 minutes, drain, and transfer to a bowl. Heat up a pan with the butter over medium heat. Add the garlic, stir, and cook for 1 minute. Add the kohlrabi slices, salt, and pepper, and cook until they are golden brown on both sides. Add the parsley, toss to coat, transfer to plates, and serve warm.

Nutrition: Calories - 87, Fat - 2. 4, Fiber - 3, Carbs - 5, Protein - 4

Turnip Fries

Preparation time: 10 minutes
Cooking time: 25 minutes
Servings: 4

Ingredients:
- 2 pounds turnips, peeled and cut into sticks
- Salt, to taste
- ¼ cup olive oil

For the seasoning mix:
- 2 tablespoons chili powder
- 1 teaspoon garlic powder
- ½ teaspoon dried oregano
- 1½ teaspoons onion powder
- 1½ tablespoons cumin

Directions:
In a bowl, mix the chili powder with the onion powder, garlic powder, cumin, and oregano, and stir well. Add the parsnips sticks, rub them well, and spread on a lined baking sheet. Season with salt, drizzle the oil, toss to coat well, and bake in the oven at 350ºF for 25 minutes. Let the parsnip fries cool before serving.

Nutrition: Calories - 140, Fat - 2, Fiber - 1, Carbs - 1, Protein - 6

Creamy Cauliflower and Spinach

Preparation time: 10 minutes
Cooking time: 15 minutes
Servings: 6

Ingredients:
- 1 cup spinach leaves
- 3 cups cauliflower florets
- ¼ cup cream
- 4 tablespoons butter
- Salt and ground black pepper, to taste
- ½ cup sour cream
- 1 avocado, pitted and peeled

Directions:
In a heatproof bowl, mix the spinach with cauliflower florets, place in a microwave, and cook for 15 minutes. Mash the avocado with a fork and add to spinach mixture. Add salt, pepper, cream, butter, and sour cream, and blend using an immersion blender. Transfer to plates and serve.

Nutrition: Calories - 190, Fat - 16, Fiber - 7, Carbs - 3, Protein - 5

Twice-baked Zucchini

Preparation time: 10 minutes
Cooking time: 30 minutes
Servings: 4

Ingredients:
- 2 zucchini, cut into half and each half in half lengthwise
- ¼ cup onion, peeled and chopped
- ½ cup cheddar cheese, shredded
- 4 bacon strips, cooked and crumbled
- ¼ cup sour cream
- 2 ounces cream cheese, softened
- 1 tablespoon jalapeño pepper, chopped
- Salt and ground black pepper, to taste
- 2 tablespoons butter

Directions:
Scoop the zucchini insides, place flesh in a bowl, and arrange the zucchini cups in a baking dish. Add the onion, cheddar cheese, crumbled bacon, jalapeño, salt, pepper, sour cream, cream cheese, and butter to the bowl. Whisk well, fill the zucchini quarters with this mixture, place in an oven at 350ºF, and bake for 30 minutes. Divide zucchini on plates, and serve.

Nutrition: Calories - 260, Fat - 22, Fiber - 4, Carbs - 3, Protein - 10

Sausage Gravy

Preparation time: 10 minutes
Cooking time: 10 minutes
Servings: 4

Ingredients:
- 4 ounces sausages, chopped
- Salt and ground black pepper, to taste
- 1 cup heavy cream
- 2 tablespoons butter
- ½ teaspoon guar gum

Directions:
Heat up a pan over medium heat, add the sausage pieces, stir, cook for 4 minutes, and transfer to a plate. Return the pan to the heat, add the butter, and melt it. Add the cream, salt, pepper, and guar gum, stir and cook until it begins to thicken. Return the sausage to pan, stir well, take off the heat, and serve.

Nutrition: Calories - 345, Fat - 34, Fiber - 0, Carbs - 2, Protein - 4

Mushroom and Hemp Pilaf

Preparation time: 10 minutes
Cooking time: 20 minutes
Servings: 4

Ingredients:
- 2 tablespoons butter
- ¼ cup almonds, sliced
- 3 mushrooms, chopped
- 1 cup hemp seeds
- Salt and ground black pepper, to taste
- ½ teaspoon garlic powder
- ½ cup chicken stock
- ¼ teaspoon dried parsley

Directions:
Heat up a pan with the butter over medium heat, add the almonds and mushrooms, stir, and cook for 4 minutes. Add the hemp seeds and stir. Add the salt, pepper, parsley, garlic powder, and stock, stir, reduce the heat, cover the pan, and simmer until the stock is absorbed. Divide on plates and serve.

Nutrition: Calories - 324, Fat - 24, Fiber - 15, Carbs - 2, Protein - 15

Asian Side Salad

Preparation time: 30 minutes
Cooking time: 10 minutes
Servings: 4

Ingredients:
- 1 cucumber, sliced thin
- 1 green onion, peeled and chopped
- 2 tablespoons coconut oil
- 1 packet Asian noodles
- 1 tablespoon balsamic vinegar
- 1 tablespoon sesame oil
- ¼ teaspoon red pepper flakes
- Salt and ground black pepper, to taste
- 1 teaspoon sesame seeds

Directions:
Cook the noodles according to package instructions, drain, and rinse well. Heat up a pan with the coconut oil over medium-high heat, add the noodles, cover pan, and fry them for 5 minutes until they are crispy.
Transfer the noodles to paper towels and drain the grease. In a bowl, mix the cucumber slices with the green onion, pepper flakes, vinegar, sesame oil, sesame seeds, salt, pepper, and noodles. Toss to coat well, keep in the refrigerator for 30 minutes, and serve.

Nutrition: Calories - 400, Fat - 34, Fiber - 2, Carbs - 4, Protein - 2

Mixed Vegetable Dish

Preparation time: 10 minutes
Cooking time: 10 minutes
Servings: 4

Ingredients:
- 14 ounces mushrooms, sliced
- 3 ounces broccoli florets
- 3.5 ounces sugar snap peas
- 6 tablespoons olive oil
- Salt and ground black pepper, to taste
- 3 ounces bell pepper, seeded and cut into strips
- 3 ounces spinach, torn
- 2 tablespoons garlic, minced
- 2 tablespoons pumpkin seeds
- A pinch of red pepper flakes

Directions:
Heat up a pan with the oil over medium-high heat, add the garlic, stir, and cook for 1 minute. Add the mushrooms, stir, and cook for 3 minutes. Add the broccoli, and stir. Add the snap peas and peppers, and stir again. Add the salt, pepper, pumpkin seeds, and pepper flakes, stir, and cook for a few minutes. Add the spinach, stir gently, cook for a couple of minutes, divide on plates, and serve.

Nutrition: Calories - 247, Fat - 23, Fiber - 4, Carbs - 3, Protein - 7

Cauliflower Polenta

Preparation time: 10 minutes
Cooking time: 1 hour
Servings: 2

Ingredients:
- 1 cauliflower head, separated into florets and chopped
- ¼ cup hazelnuts
- 1 tablespoon olive oil + 2 teaspoons extra virgin olive oil
- 1 onion, peeled and chopped
- 3 cups shiitake mushrooms, chopped
- 4 garlic cloves, peeled
- 3 tablespoons nutritional yeast
- ½ cup water
- Parsley, chopped, for serving

Directions:
Spread the hazelnuts on a lined baking sheet, place in an oven at 350°F, and bake for 10 minutes. Take the hazelnuts out of the oven, leave them to cool down, chop, and set aside. Spread the cauliflower florets on the baking sheet, drizzle 1 teaspoon oil, place in an oven at 400°F, and bake for 30 minutes. In a bowl, mix the oil with ½ teaspoon oil, and toss to coat. Put the garlic cloves on an aluminum foil, drizzle with ½ teaspoon oil, and wrap. Spread the onion next to cauliflower and garlic on the baking sheet, place in an oven everything, and bake for 20 minutes. Heat up a pan with the rest of the oil over medium-high heat, add the mushrooms, stir, and cook for 8 minutes. Take the cauliflower out of the oven and transfer to a food processor. Unwrap the garlic, peel, and add to the food processor. Add the onion, yeast, salt, and pepper, and blend well. Divide the polenta on plates, top with mushrooms, hazelnuts, and parsley, and serve.

Nutrition: Calories - 342, Fat - 21, Fiber - 12, Carbs - 3, Protein - 14

Sausage Stuffing

Preparation time: 10 minutes
Cooking time: 4 hours and 20 minutes
Servings: 8

Ingredients:
- 2 cups almond flour
- 2 tablespoons whey protein powder
- ¼ cup coconut flour
- ½ teaspoon garlic powder
- 2 teaspoons baking powder
- 1¼ cups cheddar cheese, shredded
- 2 eggs
- ¼ cup melted butter
- ¾ cup water
- ½ cup onion, peeled and chopped
- 2 tablespoons butter
- 1 red bell pepper, seeded and chopped
- 1 jalapeño pepper, chopped
- Salt and ground black pepper, to taste
- 12 ounces sausage, chopped
- 2 eggs
- ¾ cup chicken stock
- ¼ cup whipping cream

For the stuffing:

Directions:
In a bowl, mix the coconut flour with the whey protein, almond flour, garlic powder, baking powder, and 1 cup cheddar cheese, and stir. Add the water, 2 eggs, ¼ cup butter, and stir well. Transfer this to a greased baking pan, sprinkle the rest of the cheddar cheese, place in an oven at 325°F, and bake for 30 minutes. Let the bread to cool down for 15 minutes, and cube it. Spread bread cubes on a lined baking sheet, place in an oven at 200°F, and bake for 3 hours. Take bread cubes out of the oven, and set aside. Heat up a pan with 2 tablespoons butter over medium heat, add the onion, stir, and cook for 4 minutes. Add the jalapeño and red bell pepper, stir, and cook for 5 minutes. Add the salt and pepper, stir, and transfer everything to a bowl. Heat up the same pan over medium heat, add the sausage, stir, and cook for 10 minutes. Transfer the sausage to the bowl with the vegetables, stock, bread, and stir. In a separate bowl, whisk 2 eggs with some salt, pepper, and whipping cream. Add this to the sausage and bread mixture, stir, transfer to a greased baking pan, place in an oven at 325°F, and bake for 30 minutes. Serve hot.

Nutrition: Calories - 340, Fat - 4, Fiber - 6, Carbs - 3. 4, Protein - 7

Baby Mushrooms

Preparation time: 10 minutes
Cooking time: 30 minutes
Servings: 4

Ingredients:
- 4 tablespoons butter
- 16 ounces baby mushrooms
- Salt and ground black pepper, to taste
- 3 tablespoons dried onion flakes
- 3 tablespoons dried parsley
- 1 teaspoon garlic powder

Directions:
In a bowl, mix the parsley flakes with onion, salt, pepper, and garlic powder, and stir. In another bowl, mix the mushroom with melted butter and toss to coat. Add the seasoning mixture, toss well, spread on a lined baking sheet, place in an oven at 300°F, bake for 30 minutes, and serve.

Nutrition: Calories - 152, Fat - 12, Fiber - 5, Carbs - 6, Protein - 4

Green Beans with Vinaigrette

Preparation time: 10 minutes
Cooking time: 12 minutes
Serving: 8

Ingredients:
- 2 ounces chorizo, chopped
- 1 garlic clove, peeled and minced
- 1 teaspoon lemon juice
- 2 teaspoons smoked paprika
- ½ cup coconut vinegar
- 4 tablespoons macadamia nut oil
- ¼ teaspoon coriander
- Salt and ground black pepper, to taste
- 2 tablespoons coconut oil
- 2 tablespoons beef stock
- 2 pound green beans

Directions:
In a blender, mix the chorizo with salt, pepper, vinegar, garlic, lemon juice, paprika, and coriander, and pulse well. Add the stock and the macadamia nut oil and blend again. Heat up a pan with the coconut oil over medium heat, add the green beans and chorizo mixture, stir, and cook for 10 minutes. Divide on plates and serve.

Nutrition: Calories - 160, Fat - 12, Fiber - 4, Carbs - 6, Protein - 4

Braised Asian Eggplant

Preparation time: 10 minutes
Cooking time: 15 minutes
Servings: 4

Ingredients:
- 1 Asian eggplant, cut into medium-sized pieces
- 1 onion, peeled and sliced thin
- 2 tablespoon vegetable oil
- 2 teaspoons garlic, minced
- ½ cup Vietnamese sauce
- ½ cup water
- 2 teaspoons chili paste
- ¼ cup coconut milk
- 4 green onions, chopped

For the Vietnamese sauce:
- 1 teaspoon palm sugar
- ½ cup chicken stock
- 2 tablespoons fish sauce

Directions:
Put stock in a pan, and heat up over medium heat. Add the sugar, and fish sauce, stir well, and set aside. Heat up a pan over medium-high heat, add the eggplant pieces, brown them for 2 minutes, and transfer to a plate. Heat up the pan again with the oil over medium-high heat, add the onion and garlic, stir, and cook for 2 minutes. Return the eggplant pieces and cook for 2 minutes. Add the water, Vietnamese sauce, chili paste, and coconut milk, stir, and cook for 5 minutes. Add the green onions, stir, cook for 1 minute, transfer to plates, and serve.

Nutrition: Calories - 142, Fat - 7, Fiber - 4, Carbs - 5, Protein - 3

Cheddar Soufflés

Preparation time: 10 minutes
Cooking time: 25 minutes
Servings: 8

Ingredients:
- ¾ cup heavy cream
- 2 cups cheddar cheese, shredded
- 6 eggs
- Salt and ground black pepper, to taste
- ¼ teaspoon cream of tartar
- A pinch of cayenne pepper
- ½ teaspoon xanthan gum
- 1 teaspoon dry mustard
- ¼ cup fresh chives, chopped
- ½ cup almond flour
- Vegetable oil cooking spray

Directions:
In a bowl, mix the almond flour with salt, pepper, mustard, xanthan gum, and cayenne, and whisk. Add the cheese, cream, chives, eggs, and cream of tartar, and whisk again. Grease 8 ramekins with cooking spray, pour the cheddar and chives mixture, place in an oven at 350°F, bake for 25 minutes, and serve.

Nutrition: Calories - 288, Fat - 23, Fiber - 1, Carbs - 3. 3, Protein – 14

Cauliflower Side Salad

Preparation time: 10 minutes
Cooking time: 5 minutes
Servings: 10

Ingredients:

- 21 ounces cauliflower, separated into florets
- Salt and ground black pepper, to taste
- 1 cup onion, chopped
- 1 cup celery, chopped
- 2 tablespoons cider vinegar
- 1 teaspoon sucralose
- 4 eggs, hard-boiled, peeled, and chopped
- 1 cup mayonnaise
- 1 tablespoon water

Directions:

Put the cauliflower florets in a heatproof bowl, add the water, cover, and cook in a microwave for 5 minutes.
Set aside for 5 minutes and transfer to a salad bowl. Add the celery, eggs, and onions, and stir gently. In a bowl, mix the mayonnaise with salt, pepper, sucralose, and vinegar, and whisk. Add this to the salad, toss to coat well, and serve.

Nutrition: Calories - 211, Fat - 20, Fiber - 2, Carbs - 3, Protein - 4

Rice with Cauliflower

Preparation time: 10 minutes
Cooking time: 30 minutes
Servings: 4

Ingredients:

- 1 cauliflower head, separated into florets
- Salt and ground black pepper, to taste
- 10 ounces coconut milk
- ½ cup water
- 2 ginger slices
- 2 tablespoons coconut shreds, toasted

Directions:

Put the cauliflower in a food processor and blend. Transfer the cauliflower rice to a kitchen towel, press well, and set aside. Heat up a pot with the coconut milk over medium heat. Add the water and ginger, stir, and bring to a simmer. Add the cauliflower, stir, and cook for 30 minutes. Discard the ginger, add salt, pepper, and coconut shreds, stir gently, divide on plates, and serve.

Nutrition: Calories - 108, Fat - 3, Fiber - 6, Carbs - 5, Protein - 9

Ketogenic Snacks and Appetizers Recipes

Marinated Eggs

Preparation time: 2 hours and 10 minutes
Cooking time: 7 minutes
Servings: 4

Ingredients:
- 6 eggs
- 1¼ cups water
- ¼ cup unsweetened rice vinegar
- 2 tablespoons coconut aminos
- Salt and ground black pepper, to taste
- 2 garlic cloves, peeled and minced
- 1 teaspoon stevia
- 4 ounces cream cheese
- 1 tablespoon fresh chives, chopped

Directions:
Put the eggs in a pot, add the water to cover, bring to a boil over medium heat, cover, and cook for 7 minutes. Rinse the eggs with cold water, and set them aside to cool down. In a bowl, mix 1 cup water with the coconut aminos, vinegar, stevia, and garlic, and whisk. Put the eggs in this mixture, cover with a kitchen towel, and set aside for 2 hours, rotating them from time to time. Peel the eggs, cut in half, and put the egg yolks in a bowl. Add the remaining water, cream cheese, salt, pepper, and chives, and stir well. Stuff the egg whites with this mixture and serve.

Nutrition: Calories - 210, Fat - 3, Fiber - 1, Carbs - 3, Protein - 12

Sausage and Cheese Dip ✓

Preparation time: 10 minutes
Cooking time: 2 hours and 10 minutes
Servings: 28

Ingredients:
- 8 ounces cream cheese
- A pinch of salt, and black pepper
- 16 ounces sour cream
- 8 ounces pepper jack cheese, chopped
- 15 ounces canned tomatoes mixed with habaneros
- 1 pound Italian sausage, ground
- ¼ cup green onions, chopped

Directions:
Heat up a pan over medium heat, add the sausage, stir, and cook until it browns. Add the tomatoes mixture, stir, and cook for 4 minutes. Add a pinch of salt and pepper, and the green onions, stir, and cook for 4 minutes. Spread the pepper jack cheese on the bottom of a slow cooker. Add the cream cheese, sausage mixture, and sour cream, cover, and cook on high for 2 hours. Uncover the slow cooker, stir the dip, transfer to a bowl, and serve.

Nutrition: Calories - 144, Fat - 12, Fiber - 1, Carbs - 3, Protein - 6

Onion and Cauliflower Dip ✓

Preparation time: 2 hours 10 minutes
Cooking time: 30 minutes
Servings: 24

Ingredients:
- 1½ cups chicken stock
- 1 cauliflower head, separated into florets
- ¼ cup mayonnaise
- ½ cup onion, peeled and chopped
- ¾ cup cream cheese
- ½ teaspoon chili powder
- ½ teaspoon cumin
- ½ teaspoon garlic powder
- Salt and ground black pepper, to taste

Directions:
Put the stock in a pot, add the cauliflower and onion, heat up over medium heat, and cook for 30 minutes. Add the chili powder, salt, pepper, cumin, and garlic powder, and stir. Add cream cheese, and stir a bit until it melts. Blend using an immersion blender and mix with the mayonnaise. Transfer to a bowl, and keep in the refrigerator for 2 hours before serving.

Nutrition: Calories - 60, Fat - 4, Fiber - 1, Carbs - 1, Protein - 1

Pesto Crackers

Preparation time: 10 minutes
Cooking time: 17 minutes
Servings: 6

Ingredients:
- ½ teaspoon baking powder
- Salt and ground black pepper, to taste
- 1¼ cups almond flour
- ¼ teaspoon dried basil
- 1 garlic clove, peeled and minced
- 2 tablespoons basil pesto
- A pinch of cayenne pepper
- 3 tablespoons butter

Directions:
In a bowl, mix the salt, pepper, baking powder, and almond flour. Add the garlic, cayenne, and basil, and stir. Add the pesto and whisk. Add butter and mix the dough with your fingers. Spread this dough on a lined baking sheet, place in an oven at 325ºF, and bake for 17 minutes. Set aside to cool down, cut the crackers, and serve.

Nutrition: Calories - 200, Fat - 20, Fiber - 1, Carbs - 4, Protein - 7

Pumpkin Muffins

Preparation time: 10 minutes
Cooking time: 15 minutes
Servings: 18

Ingredients:
- ¼ cup sunflower seed butter
- ¾ cup pumpkin puree
- 2 tablespoons flaxseed meal
- ¼ cup coconut flour
- ½ cup erythritol
- ½ teaspoon ground nutmeg
- 1 teaspoon ground cinnamon
- ½ teaspoon baking soda
- 1 egg
- ½ teaspoon baking powder
- A pinch of salt

Directions:
In a bowl, mix the butter with the pumpkin puree, and egg and blend well. Add the flaxseed meal, coconut flour, erythritol, baking soda, baking powder, nutmeg, cinnamon, and a pinch of salt and stir well. Spoon this into a greased muffin pan, place in an oven at 350ºF, and bake for 15 minutes. Let the muffins to cool down and serve.

Nutrition: Calories - 50, Fat - 3, Fiber - 1, Carbs - 2, Protein - 2

Special Tortilla Chips

Preparation time: 10 minutes
Cooking time: 14 minutes
Servings: 6

Ingredients:
For the tortillas:
- 2 teaspoons olive oil
- 1 cup flaxseed meal
- 2 tablespoons psyllium husk powder
- ¼ teaspoon xanthan gum
- 1 cup water
- ½ teaspoon curry powder
- 3 teaspoons coconut flour

For the chips:
- 6 flaxseed tortillas
- Salt and ground black pepper, to taste
- 3 tablespoons vegetable oil
- Fresh salsa, for serving
- Sour cream, for serving

Directions:
In a bowl, mix the flaxseed meal with the psyllium powder, olive oil, xanthan gum, water, and curry powder, and mix until you obtain an elastic dough. Spread coconut flour on a working surface. Divide the dough into 6 pieces, place each piece on the work surface, roll into a circle, and cut each into 6 pieces. Heat up a pan with the vegetable oil over medium-high heat, add the tortilla chips, cook for 2 minutes on each side, and transfer to paper towels. Put the tortilla chips in a bowl, season with salt, and pepper, and serve with some fresh salsa, and sour cream on the side.

Nutrition: Calories - 30, Fat - 3, Fiber - 1. 2, Carbs - 0. 5, Protein - 1

Jalapeño Balls

Preparation time: 10 minutes
Cooking time: 10 minutes
Servings: 3

Ingredients:
- 3 bacon slices
- 3 ounces cream cheese
- ¼ teaspoon onion powder
- Salt and ground black pepper, to taste
- 1 jalapeño pepper, chopped
- ½ teaspoon dried parsley
- ¼ teaspoon garlic powder

Directions:
Heat up a pan over medium-high heat, add the bacon, cook until crispy, transfer to paper towels, drain grease, and crumble. Reserve the bacon fat from the pan. In a bowl, mix the cream cheese with the jalapeño pepper, onion powder, garlic powder, parsley, salt, and pepper, and stir well. Add the bacon fat and crumbled bacon, stir gently, shape balls from this mixture, and serve.

Nutrition: Calories - 200, Fat - 18, Fiber - 1, Carbs - 2, Protein - 5

Pepperoni Bombs

Preparation time: 10 minutes
Cooking time: 0 minutes
Servings: 6

Ingredients:
- 8 black olives, pitted and chopped
- Salt and ground black pepper, to taste
- 2 tablespoons sundried tomato pesto
- 14 pepperoni slices, chopped
- 4 ounces cream cheese
- 1 tablespoons fresh basil, chopped

Directions:
In a bowl, mix the cream cheese with salt, pepper, pepperoni, basil, sundried tomato pesto, and black olives, and stir well. Shape balls from this mixture, arrange on a platter, and serve.

Nutrition: Calories - 110, Fat - 10, Fiber - 0, Carbs - 1. 4, Protein - 3

Cheeseburger Muffins

Preparation time: 10 minutes
Cooking time: 30 minutes
Servings: 9

Ingredients:
- ½ cup flaxseed meal
- ½ cup almond flour
- Salt and ground black pepper, to taste
- 2 eggs
- 1 teaspoon baking powder
- ¼ cups sour cream

For the filling:
- ½ teaspoon onion powder
- 16 ounces ground beef
- Salt and ground black pepper, to taste
- 2 tablespoons tomato paste
- ½ teaspoon garlic powder
- ½ cup cheddar cheese, grated
- 2 tablespoons mustard

Directions:
In a bowl, mix the almond flour with flaxseed meal, salt, pepper, and baking powder, and whisk. Add the eggs, and sour cream, and stir well. Divide this into a greased muffin pan and press well using your fingers. Heat up a pan over medium-high heat, add the beef, stir, and brown for a few minutes. Add the salt, pepper, onion powder, garlic powder, and tomato paste, and stir well. Cook for 5 minutes, and take off the heat. Fill the cupcakes crusts with this mixture, place in an oven at 350ºF, and bake for 15 minutes. Spread the cheese on top, place in an oven again, and bake muffins for 5 minutes. Serve warm.

Nutrition: Calories - 245, Fat - 16, Fiber - 6, Carbs - 2, Protein - 14

Pizza Dip

Preparation time: 10 minutes
Cooking time: 20 minutes
Servings: 4

Ingredients:
- 4 ounces cream cheese, softened
- ½ cup mozzarella cheese
- ¼ cup sour cream
- Salt and ground black pepper, to taste
- ½ cup tomato sauce
- ¼ cup mayonnaise
- ¼ cup Parmesan cheese, grated
- 1 tablespoon green bell pepper, seeded and chopped
- 6 pepperoni slices, chopped
- ½ teaspoon Italian seasoning
- 4 black olives, pitted and chopped

Directions:
In a bowl, mix the cream cheese with the mozzarella cheese, sour cream, mayonnaise, salt, and pepper, and stir well. Spread this into 4 ramekins, add a layer of tomato sauce, then layer Parmesan cheese, and top with bell pepper, pepperoni, Italian seasoning, and black olives. Place in an oven at 350ºF and bake for 20 minutes. Serve warm.

Nutrition: Calories - 400, Fat - 34, Fiber - 4, Carbs - 4, Protein - 15

Flaxseed and Almond Muffins

Preparation time: 10 minutes
Cooking time: 15 minutes
Servings: 20

Ingredients:
- ½ cup flaxseed meal
- ½ cup almond flour
- 3 tablespoons swerve
- 1 tablespoon psyllium powder
- A pinch of salt
- Vegetable oil cooking spray
- ¼ teaspoon baking powder
- 1 egg
- ¼ cup coconut milk
- ⅓ cup sour cream
- 4 hot dogs, cut into 20 pieces

Directions:
In a bowl, mix the flaxseed meal with flour, psyllium powder, swerve, salt, and baking powder, and stir. Add the egg, sour cream, and coconut milk, and whisk. Grease a muffin tray with cooking oil, divide the batter you've just make, stick a hot dog piece in the middle of each muffin, place in an oven at 350ºF, and bake for 12 minutes. Broil in preheated broil for 3 minutes, divide on a platter, and serve.

Nutrition: Calories - 80, Fat - 6, Fiber - 1, Carbs - 1, Protein - 3

Fried Queso

Preparation time: 10 minutes
Cooking time: 10 minutes
Servings: 6

Ingredients:
- 2 ounces olives, pitted and chopped
- 5 ounces queso blanco, cubed and slightly frozen
- A pinch of red pepper flakes
- 1½ tablespoons olive oil

Directions:
Heat up a pan with the oil over medium-high heat, add the queso cubes, and cook until the bottom melts a bit. Flip the cubes with a spatula, and sprinkle black olives on top. Let the cubes to cook a bit more, flip again, sprinkle with red pepper flakes, and cook until crispy. Flip, cook on the other side until crispy as well, transfer to a cutting board, cut into small blocks, and serve.

Nutrition: Calories - 500, Fat - 43, Fiber - 4, Carbs - 2, Protein - 30

Maple and Pecan Bars

Preparation time: 10 minutes
Cooking time: 25 minutes
Servings: 12

Ingredients:
- ½ cup flaxseed meal
- 2 cups pecans, toasted, and crushed
- 1 cup almond flour
- ½ cup coconut oil
- ¼ teaspoon stevia
- ½ cup coconut, shredded
- ¼ cup "maple syrup"

For the maple syrup:
- ¼ cup erythritol
- 2¼ teaspoons coconut oil
- 1 tablespoon butter
- ¼ teaspoon xanthan gum
- ¾ cup water
- 2 teaspoons maple extract
- ½ teaspoon vanilla extract

Directions:
In a heatproof bowl, mix the butter with 2¼ teaspoons coconut oil, and xanthan gum, stir, place in a microwave, and heat up for 1 minute. Add the erythritol, water, maple, and vanilla extract, stir well, and heat up in the microwave for 1 minute. In a bowl, mix the flaxseed meal with coconut and almond flour, and stir. Add the pecans and stir again. Add the ¼ cup "maple syrup," stevia, and ½ cup coconut oil, and stir well. Spread this in a baking dish, press well, place in an oven at 350°F, and bake for 25 minutes. Set aside to cool down, cut into 12 bars, and serve.

Nutrition: Calories - 300, Fat - 30, Fiber - 12, Carbs - 2, Protein - 5

Baked Chia Seeds

Preparation time: 10 minutes
Cooking time: 35 minutes
Servings: 36

Ingredients:
- 1¼ cup ice water
- ½ cup chia seeds, ground
- 3 ounces cheddar, cheese, grated
- ¼ teaspoon xanthan gum
- 2 tablespoons olive oil
- 2 tablespoons psyllium husk powder
- ¼ teaspoon dried oregano
- ¼ teaspoon garlic powder
- ¼ teaspoon onion powder
- Salt and ground black pepper, to taste
- ¼ teaspoon sweet paprika

Directions:
In a bowl, mix the chia seeds with the xanthan gum, psyllium powder, oregano, garlic, and onion powder, paprika, salt, and pepper, and stir. Add the oil and stir well. Add the ice water and stir until you obtain a firm dough. Spread this on a baking sheet, place in an oven at 350°F, and bake for 35 minutes. Set aside to cool down, cut into 36 crackers, and serve.

Nutrition: Calories - 50, Fat - 3, Fiber - 1, Carbs - 0. 1, Protein - 2

Simple Tomato Tarts

Preparation time: 10 minutes
Cooking time: 1 hour and 10 minutes
Servings: 12

Ingredients:
- ¼ cup olive oil
- 2 tomatoes, cored and sliced
- Salt and ground black pepper, to taste

For the base:
- 5 tablespoons butter
- 1 tablespoon psyllium husk
- ½ cup almond flour
- 2 tablespoons coconut flour
- A pinch of salt

For the filling:
- 2 teaspoons garlic, minced
- 3 teaspoons fresh thyme, chopped
- 2 tablespoons olive oil
- 3 ounces goat cheese, crumbled
- 1 small onion, sliced thin

Directions:
Spread tomato slices on a lined baking sheet, season with salt, and pepper, drizzle ¼ cup olive oil, place in an oven at 425ºF, and bake for 40 minutes. In a food processor, mix the almond flour with the psyllium husk, coconut flour, salt, pepper, and cold butter, and stir until you obtain a dough. Divide this dough into silicone cupcake molds, press well, place in an oven at 350ºF, and bake for 20 minutes. Take the cupcakes out of the oven and set aside. Take the tomato slices out of the oven and let them cool briefly. Divide the tomato slices on top of cupcakes. Heat up a pan with 2 tablespoons olive oil over medium-high heat, add the onion, stir, and cook for 4 minutes. Add the garlic and thyme, stir, cook for 1 minute, and take off the heat. Spread this mixture on top of tomato slices. Sprinkle with goat cheese, place in an oven again, and cook at 350ºF for 5 minutes. Arrange on a platter and serve.

Nutrition: Calories - 163, Fat - 13, Fiber - 1, Carbs - 3, Protein - 3

Avocado Dip

Preparation time: 3 hours and 10 minutes
Cooking time: 10 minutes
Servings: 4

Ingredients:
- ¼ cup erythritol powder
- 2 avocados, pitted, peeled, and cut into slices
- ¼ teaspoon stevia
- ½ cup fresh cilantro, chopped
- Juice, and zest of 2 limes
- 1 cup coconut milk

Directions:
Place the avocado slices on a lined baking sheet, squeeze half of the lime juice over them, and keep in a freezer for 3 hours. Heat up the coconut milk in a pan over medium heat. Add the lime zest, stir, and bring to a boil. Add the erythritol powder, stir, take off the heat, and set aside to cool. Transfer the avocado to a food processor, add the rest of the lime juice, and the cilantro, and pulse well. Add the coconut milk mixture, and stevia, and blend well. Transfer to a bowl and serve.

Nutrition: Calories - 150, Fat - 14, Fiber - 2, Carbs - 4, Protein - 2

Prosciutto-wrapped Shrimp

Preparation time: 10 minutes
Cooking time: 20 minutes
Servings: 16

Ingredients:
- 2 tablespoons olive oil
- 10 ounces already cooked shrimp, peeled and deveined
- 1 tablespoons fresh mint, chopped
- 2 tablespoons erythritol
- ⅓ cup blackberries, mashed
- 11 prosciutto sliced
- ⅓ cup red wine

Directions:
Wrap each shrimp in prosciutto slices, arrange on a lined baking sheet, drizzle the olive oil over them, place in an oven at 425ºF, and bake for 15 minutes. Heat up a pan with mashed blackberries over medium heat, add the mint, wine, and erythritol, stir, cook for 3 minutes, and take off the heat. Arrange shrimp on a platter, drizzle blackberries sauce over them, and serve.

Nutrition: Calories - 245, Fat - 12, Fiber - 2, Carbs - 1, Protein - 14

Broccoli and Cheddar Biscuits

Preparation time: 10 minutes
Cooking time: 25 minutes
Servings: 12

Ingredients:
- 4 cups broccoli florets
- 1½ cup almond flour
- 1 teaspoon paprika
- Salt and ground black pepper, to taste
- 2 eggs
- ¼ cup coconut oil
- 2 cups cheddar cheese, grated
- 1 teaspoon garlic powder
- ½ teaspoon apple cider vinegar
- ½ teaspoon baking soda

Directions:
Put the broccoli florets in a food processor, add the some salt and pepper, and blend well. In a bowl, mix the almond flour with salt, pepper, paprika, garlic powder, and baking soda, and stir. Add the cheddar cheese, coconut oil, eggs, and vinegar, and stir. Add the broccoli, and stir again. Shape 12 patties, arrange on a baking sheet, place in an oven at 375ºF, and bake for 20 minutes. Turn the oven to broiler, and broil the biscuits for 5 minutes. Arrange on a platter and serve.

Nutrition: Calories - 163, Fat - 12, Fiber - 2, Carbs - 2, Protein - 7

Corndogs

Preparation time: 10 minutes
Cooking time: 10 minutes
Servings: 4

Ingredients:
- 1½ cups olive oil
- 2 tablespoons heavy cream
- 1 cup almond meal
- 4 sausages
- 1 teaspoon baking powder
- 1 teaspoon Italian seasoning
- 2 eggs
- ½ teaspoon turmeric
- Salt and ground black pepper, to taste
- A pinch of cayenne pepper

Directions:
In a bowl, mix the almond meal with the Italian seasoning, baking powder, turmeric, salt, pepper, and cayenne, and stir well. In another bowl, mix the eggs with heavy cream, and whisk. Combine the 2 mixtures and stir well. Dip sausages in this mixture, and place them on a plate. Heat up a pan with the oil over medium-high heat, add the sausages, cook for 2 minutes on each side, and transfer to paper towels. Drain grease, arrange on a platter, and serve.

Nutrition: Calories - 345, Fat - 33, Fiber - 4, Carbs - 5, Protein - 16

Mini Bell Pepper Nachos

Preparation time: 10 minutes
Cooking time: 20 minutes
Servings: 6

Ingredients:
- 1 pound mini bell peppers, seeded and cut into halves
- Salt and ground black pepper, to taste
- 1 teaspoon garlic powder
- 1 teaspoon sweet paprika
- ½ teaspoon dried oregano
- ¼ teaspoon red pepper flakes
- 1 pound ground beef
- 1½ cups cheddar cheese, shredded
- 1 tablespoons chili powder
- 1 teaspoon cumin
- ½ cup tomato, cored and chopped
- Sour cream, for serving

Directions:
In a bowl, mix the chili powder with paprika, salt, pepper, cumin, oregano, pepper flakes, and garlic powder, and stir. Heat up a pan over medium heat, add the beef, stir, and brown for 10 minutes. Add the chili powder mixture, stir, and take off the heat. Arrange pepper halves on a lined baking sheet, stuff them with the beef mixture, sprinkle with the cheese, place in an oven at 400ºF, and bake for 10 minutes. Take the peppers out of the oven, sprinkle with the tomatoes, divide on plates, and serve with sour cream on top.

Nutrition: Calories - 350, Fat - 22, Fiber - 3, Carbs - 6, Protein - 27

Almond Butter Bars

Preparation time: 2 hours and 10 minutes
Cooking time: 2 minutes
Servings: 12

Ingredients:
- ¾ cup coconut, unsweetened and shredded
- ¾ cup almond butter
- ¾ cup stevia
- 1 cup almond butter
- 2 tablespoons almond butter
- 4. 5 ounces dark chocolate, chopped
- 2 tablespoons coconut oil

Directions:
In a bowl, mix the almond flour with stevia and coconut, and stir well. Heat up a pan over medium-low heat, add the 1 cup almond butter and coconut oil, and whisk. Add this to almond flour and stir well. Transfer this to a baking dish and press well. Heat up another pan with the chocolate, stirring often. Add the rest of the almond butter and whisk again. Pour this over almond mixture, and spread evenly. Place in the refrigerator for 2 hours, cut into 12 bars, and serve.

Nutrition: Calories - 140, Fat - 2, Fiber - 1, Carbs - 5, Protein - 1

Saucy Zucchini

Preparation time: 10 minutes
Cooking time: 15 minutes
Servings: 4

Ingredients:
- 1 cup mozzarella cheese, shredded
- ¼ cup tomato sauce
- 1 zucchini, sliced
- Salt and ground black pepper, to taste
- A pinch of cumin
- Vegetable oil cooking spray

Directions:
Spray a cooking sheet with some oil and arrange zucchini slices on it. Spread the tomato sauce all over the zucchini slices, season with salt, pepper, and cumin, and sprinkle with shredded mozzarella. Place in an oven at 350ºF and bake for 15 minutes. Arrange on a platter, and serve.

Nutrition: Calories - 140, Fat - 4, Fiber - 2, Carbs - 6, Protein - 4

Zucchini Chips

Preparation time: 10 minutes
Cooking time: 3 hours
Servings: 8

Ingredients:
- 3 zucchini, sliced thin
- Salt and ground black pepper, to taste
- 2 tablespoons olive oil
- 2 tablespoons balsamic vinegar

Directions:
In a bowl, mix the oil with vinegar, salt, and pepper, and whisk. Add the zucchini slices, toss to coat well, and spread on a lined baking sheet, place in an oven at 200ºF, and bake for 3 hours. Let the chips to cool down and serve.

Nutrition: Calories - 40, Fat - 3, Fiber - 7, Carbs - 3, Protein - 7

Simple Hummus

Preparation time: 10 minutes
Cooking time: 0 minutes
Servings: 5

Ingredients:
- 4 cups zucchini, diced
- ¼ cup olive oil
- Salt and ground black pepper, to taste
- 4 garlic cloves, peeled and minced
- ¾ cup tahini
- ½ cup lemon juice
- 1 tablespoon cumin

Directions:
In a blender, mix the zucchini with salt, pepper, oil, lemon juice, garlic, tahini, and cumin, and blend well. Transfer to a bowl and serve.

Nutrition: Calories - 80, Fat - 5, Fiber - 3, Carbs - 6, Protein - 7

Celery Sticks

Preparation time: 10 minutes
Cooking time: 0 minutes
Servings: 12

Ingredients:
- 2 cups rotisserie chicken, shredded
- 6 celery stalks, cut into halves
- 3 tablespoons tomato sauce
- ¼ cup mayonnaise
- Salt and ground black pepper, to taste
- ½ teaspoon garlic powder
- Some chopped chives, for serving

Directions:
In a bowl, mix the chicken with salt, pepper, garlic powder, mayonnaise, and tomato sauce, and stir well. Arrange the celery pieces on a platter, spread the chicken mixture over them, sprinkle some chives, and serve.

Nutrition: Calories - 100, Fat - 2, Fiber - 3, Carbs - 1, Protein - 6

Beef Jerky

Preparation time: 6 hours
Cooking time: 4 hours
Servings: 6

Ingredients:
- 24 ounces amber
- 2 cups soy sauce
- ½ cup Worcestershire sauce
- 2 tablespoons black peppercorns
- 2 tablespoons ground black pepper
- 2 pounds beef round, sliced

Directions:
In a bowl, mix the soy sauce with the black peppercorns, black pepper, and Worcestershire sauce, and whisk. Add the beef slices, toss to coat, and set aside in the refrigerator for 6 hours. Spread this on a rack, place in an oven at 370ºF, and bake for 4 hours. Transfer to a bowl and serve.

Nutrition: Calories - 300, Fat - 12, Fiber - 4, Carbs - 3, Protein - 8

Crab Dip

Preparation time: 10 minutes
Cooking time: 30 minutes
Servings: 8

Ingredients:
- 8 bacon strips, sliced
- 12 ounces crab meat
- ½ cup mayonnaise
- ½ cup sour cream
- 8 ounces cream cheese
- 2 poblano pepper, seeded, and chopped
- 2 tablespoons lemon juice
- Salt and ground black pepper, to taste
- 4 garlic cloves, peeled and minced
- 4 green onions, minced
- ½ cup Parmesan cheese+ ½ cup Parmesan cheese, grated
- Salt and ground black pepper, to taste

Directions:
Heat up a pan over medium-high heat, add the bacon, cook until crispy, transfer to paper towels, chop, and set aside to cool down. In a bowl, mix the sour cream with the cream cheese and mayonnaise, and stir well. Add the ½ cup Parmesan cheese, poblano peppers, bacon, green onion, garlic, and lemon juice, and stir again. Add the crab meat, salt, and pepper, and stir gently. Pour this into a heatproof baking dish, spread the rest of the Parmesan cheese, place in an oven, bake at 350ºF for 20 minutes, and serve.

Nutrition: Calories - 200, Fat - 7, Fiber - 2, Carbs - 4, Protein - 6

Spinach Balls

Preparation time: 10 minutes
Cooking time: 12 minutes
Servings: 30

Ingredients:
- 4 tablespoons melted butter
- 2 eggs
- 1 cup almond flour
- 16 ounces spinach
- ⅓ cup feta cheese, crumbled
- ¼ teaspoon ground nutmeg
- ⅓ cup Parmesan cheese, grated
- Salt and ground black pepper, to taste
- 1 tablespoon onion powder
- 3 tablespoons whipping cream
- 1 teaspoon garlic powder

Directions:
In a blender, mix the spinach with the butter, eggs, almond flour, feta cheese, Parmesan cheese, nutmeg, whipping cream, salt, pepper, onion, and garlic pepper, and blend well. Transfer to a bowl and keep in the freezer for 10 minutes. Shape 30 spinach balls, arrange them on a lined baking sheet, place in an oven at 350ºF, and bake for 12 minutes. Let the spinach balls to cool down and serve.

Nutrition: Calories - 60, Fat - 5, Fiber - 1, Carbs - 0. 7, Protein - 2

Garlic Spinach Dip

Preparation time: 10 minutes
Cooking time: 35 minutes
Servings: 6

Ingredients:
- 6 bacon slices
- 5 ounces spinach
- ½ cup sour cream
- 8 ounces cream cheese, softened
- 1½ tablespoons fresh parsley, chopped
- 2. 5 ounces Parmesan cheese, grated
- 1 tablespoon lemon juice
- Salt and ground black pepper, to taste
- 1 tablespoon garlic, minced

Directions:
Heat up a pan over medium heat, add the bacon, cook until crispy, transfer to paper towels, drain grease, crumble, and set aside in a bowl. Heat up the same pan with the bacon grease over medium heat, add the spinach, stir, cook for 2 minutes, and transfer to a bowl. In another bowl, mix the cream cheese with garlic, salt, pepper, sour cream, and parsley, and stir well. Add the bacon and stir again. Add the lemon juice and spinach, and stir. Add the Parmesan cheese and stir again. Divide this into ramekins, place in an oven at 350ºF, and bake for 25 minutes. Turn the oven to broil and broil for 4 minutes. Serve with crackers.

Nutrition: Calories - 345, Fat - 12, Fiber - 3, Carbs - 6, Protein - 11

Stuffed Mushrooms

Preparation time: 10 minutes
Cooking time: 20 minutes
Servings: 5

Ingredients:
- ¼ cup mayonnaise
- 1 teaspoon garlic powder
- 1 onion, peeled and chopped
- 24 ounces white mushroom caps
- Salt and ground black pepper, to taste
- 1 teaspoon curry powder
- 4 ounces cream cheese, softened
- ¼ cup sour cream
- ½ cup queso blanco or Monterey Jack cheese, shredded
- 1 cup shrimp, cooked, peeled, deveined, and chopped

Directions:
In a bowl, mix the mayonnaise with the garlic powder, onion, curry powder, cream cheese, sour cream, Mexican cheese, shrimp, salt and pepper to taste, and whisk. Stuff the mushrooms with this mixture, place on a baking sheet, and cook in the oven at 350°F for 20 minutes. Arrange on a platter and serve.

Nutrition: Calories - 244, Fat - 20, Fiber - 3, Carbs - 7, Protein - 14

Breadsticks

Preparation time: 10 minutes
Cooking time: 15 minutes
Servings: 24

Ingredients:
- 3 tablespoons cream cheese, softened
- 1 tablespoon psyllium powder
- ¾ cup almond flour
- 2 cups mozzarella cheese, melted for 30 seconds in the microwave
- 1 teaspoon baking powder
- 1 egg
- 2 tablespoons Italian seasoning
- Salt and ground black pepper, to taste
- 3 ounces cheddar cheese, grated
- 1 teaspoon onion powder

Directions:
In a bowl, mix the psyllium powder with almond flour, baking powder, salt, and pepper, and whisk. Add the cream cheese, melted mozzarella cheese, and egg, and stir using your hands until you obtain a dough. Spread this on a baking sheet, and cut into 24 sticks. Sprinkle with onion powder and Italian seasoning over them. Top with cheddar cheese, place in an oven at 350°F, bake for 15 minutes, and serve.

Nutrition: Calories - 245, Fat - 12, Fiber - 5, Carbs - 3, Protein - 14

Italian Meatballs

Preparation time: 10 minutes
Cooking time: 6 minutes
Servings: 16

Ingredients:
- 1 egg
- Salt and ground black pepper, to taste
- ¼ cup almond flour
- 1 pound ground turkey
- ½ teaspoon garlic powder
- 2 tablespoons sundried tomatoes, cored and chopped
- ½ cup mozzarella cheese, shredded
- 2 tablespoons olive oil
- 2 tablespoon fresh basil, chopped

Directions:
In a bowl, mix the turkey with salt, pepper, egg, almond flour, garlic powder, sundried tomatoes, mozzarella, and basil, and stir well. Shape 12 meatballs, heat up a pan with the oil over medium-high heat, drop meatballs, and cook them for 2 minutes on each side. Arrange on a platter and serve.

Nutrition: Calories - 80, Fat - 6, Fiber - 3, Carbs - 5, Protein - 7

Parmesan Wings

Preparation time: 10 minutes
Cooking time: 24 minutes
Servings: 6

Ingredients:
- 6-pound chicken wings, cut in half
- Salt and ground black pepper, to taste
- ½ teaspoon Italian seasoning
- 2 tablespoons butter
- ½ cup Parmesan cheese, grated
- A pinch of red pepper flakes
- 1 teaspoon garlic powder
- 1 egg

Directions:
Arrange the chicken wings on a lined baking sheet, place in an oven at 425°F, and bake for 17 minutes. In a blender, mix the butter with the cheese, egg, salt, pepper, pepper flakes, garlic powder, and Italian seasoning, and blend well. Take the chicken wings out of the oven, flip them, turn oven to broil, and broil them for 5 minutes. Take the chicken pieces out of the oven again, pour sauce over them, toss to coat well, broil for 1 minute, and serve.

Nutrition: Calories - 134, Fat - 8, Fiber - 1, Carbs - 0. 5, Protein - 14

Cheese Sticks

Preparation time: 1 hour and 10 minutes
Cooking time: 20 minutes
Servings: 16

Ingredients:
- 2 eggs, whisked
- Salt and ground black pepper, to taste
- 8 mozzarella string cheese pieces, cut in half
- 1 cup Parmesan cheese, grated
- 1 tablespoon Italian seasoning
- ½ cup olive oil
- 1 garlic clove, peeled and minced

Directions:
In a bowl, mix the Parmesan cheese with salt, pepper, Italian seasoning, and garlic, and stir well. Put the whisked eggs in another bowl. Dip the mozzarella sticks in the egg mixture, then in the cheese mixture. Dip them again in the egg mixture, then in Parmesan cheese mixture, and keep them in the freezer for 1 hour. Heat up a pan with the oil over medium-high heat, add the cheese sticks, fry them until they are golden on one side, flip, and cook them the same way on the other side. Arrange them on a platter and serve.

Nutrition: Calories - 140, Fat - 5, Fiber - 1, Carbs - 3, Protein - 4

Broccoli Sticks

Preparation time: 10 minutes
Cooking time: 20 minutes
Servings: 20

Ingredients:
- 1 egg
- 2 cups broccoli florets
- ⅓ cup cheddar cheese, grated
- ¼ cup onion, peeled and chopped
- ⅓ cup panko bread crumbs
- ⅓ cup Italian bread crumbs
- 2 tablespoons fresh parsley, chopped
- A drizzle of olive oil
- Salt and ground black pepper, to taste

Directions:
Heat up a pot with water over medium heat, add the broccoli, steam for 1 minute, drain, chop, and put into a bowl. Add the egg, cheddar cheese, panko, Italian bread crumbs, salt, pepper, and parsley, and stir well. Shape sticks out of this mixture using your hands and place them on a baking sheet that you've greased with olive oil. Place in an oven at 400°F, and bake for 20 minutes. Arrange on a platter and serve.

Nutrition: Calories - 100, Fat - 4, Fiber - 2, Carbs - 7, Protein - 7

Bacon Delight

Preparation time: 15 minutes
Cooking time: 1 hour and 20 minutes
Servings: 16

Ingredients:
- ½ teaspoon ground cinnamon
- 2 tablespoons erythritol
- 16 bacon slices
- 1 tablespoon coconut oil
- 3 ounces dark chocolate
- 1 teaspoon maple extract

Directions:
In a bowl, mix the cinnamon with the erythrito and stir. Arrange the bacon slices on a lined baking sheet and sprinkle cinnamon mixture over them. Flip the bacon slices and sprinkle the cinnamon mixture over them again. Place in an oven at 275ºF and bake for 1 hour. Heat up a pot with the oil over medium heat, add the chocolate, and stir until it melts. Add the maple extract, stir, take off the heat, and set aside to cool. Take the bacon strips out of the oven, let them cool down, dip each in chocolate mixture, place them on a parchment paper, and let them cool down completely. Serve cold.

Nutrition: Calories - 150, Fat - 4, Fiber - 0. 4, Carbs - 1. 1, Protein - 3

Taco Cups

Preparation time: 10 minutes
Cooking time: 40 minutes
Servings: 30

Ingredients:
- 1 pound ground beef
- 2 cups cheddar cheese, shredded
- ¼ cup water
- Salt and ground black pepper, to taste
- 2 tablespoons cumin
- 2 tablespoons chili powder
- Pico de gallo, for serving

Directions:
Divide spoonfuls of cheddar cheese on a lined baking sheet, place in an oven at 350ºF, and bake for 7 minutes. Let the cheese to cool down for 1 minute, transfer them to mini cupcake molds, and shape them into cups. Heat up a pan over medium-high heat, add the beef, stir, and cook until it browns. Add the water, salt, pepper, cumin, and chili powder, stir, and cook for 5 minutes. Divide into cheese cups, top with pico de gallo, transfer them all to a platter, and serve.

Nutrition: Calories - 140, Fat - 6, Fiber - 0, Carbs - 6, Protein - 15

Chicken Egg Rolls

Preparation time: 2 hours and 10 minutes
Cooking time: 15 minutes
Servings: 12

Ingredients:
- 4 ounces blue cheese
- 2 cups chicken, cooked, and diced
- Salt and ground black pepper, to taste
- 2 green onions, chopped
- 2 celery stalks, diced
- ½ cup tomato sauce
- ½ teaspoon erythritol
- 12 egg roll wrappers
- Vegetable oil

Directions:
In a bowl, mix the chicken meat with the blue cheese, salt, pepper, green onions, celery, tomato sauce, and sweetener, stir well, and keep in the refrigerator for 2 hours. Place the egg wrappers on a working surface, divide chicken mixture on them, roll, and seal edges. Heat up a pan with vegetable oil over medium-high heat, add the egg rolls, cook until they are golden, flip, and cook on the other side as well. Arrange on a platter and serve them.

Nutrition: Calories - 220, Fat - 7, Fiber - 2, Carbs - 6, Protein - 10

Cheese Fries

Preparation time: 10 minutes
Cooking time: 5 minutes
Servings: 4

Ingredients:
- 1 cup marinara sauce
- 8 ounces queso blanco, patted dried, and sliced into fries
- 2 ounces tallow

Directions:
Heat up a pan with the tallow over medium-high heat. Add the halloumi pieces, cover, cook for 2 minutes on each side, and transfer to paper towels. Drain the excess grease, transfer them to a bowl, and serve with marinara sauce on the side.

Nutrition: Calories - 200, Fat - 16, Fiber - 1, Carbs - 1, Protein - 13

Jalapeño Crisps

Preparation time: 10 minutes
Cooking time: 25 minutes
Servings: 20

Ingredients:
- 3 tablespoons olive oil
- 5 jalapeños, sliced
- 8 ounces Parmesan cheese, grated
- ½ teaspoon onion powder
- Salt and ground black pepper, to taste
- Tabasco sauce, for serving

Directions:
In a bowl, mix the jalapeño slices with salt, pepper, oil, and onion powder, toss to coat, and spread on a lined baking sheet. Place in an oven at 450ºF and bake for 15 minutes. Take the jalapeño slices out of the oven, and let them cool down. In a bowl, mix the pepper slices with the cheese, and press well. Arrange all slices on another lined baking sheet, place in an oven again, and bake for 10 minutes. Let the jalapeños to cool down, arrange on a plate, and serve with Tabasco sauce on the side.

Nutrition: Calories - 50, Fat - 3, Fiber - 0. 1, Carbs - 0. 3, Protein - 2

Cucumber Cups

Preparation time: 10 minutes
Cooking time: 0 minutes
Servings: 24

Ingredients:
- 2 cucumbers, peeled, cut into ¾-inch slices, and some of the seeds scooped out
- ½ cup sour cream
- Salt, and ground white pepper, to taste
- 6 ounces smoked salmon, flaked
- ⅓ cup fresh cilantro, chopped
- 2 teaspoons lime juice
- 1 tablespoon lime zest
- A pinch of cayenne pepper

Directions:
In a bowl, mix the salmon with salt, pepper, cayenne, sour cream, lime juice, and zest, and cilantro, and stir well. Fill each cucumber cup with this salmon mixture, arrange on a platter, and serve.

Nutrition: Calories - 30, Fat - 11, Fiber - 1, Carbs - 1, Protein - 2

Caviar Salad

Preparation time: 6 minutes
Cooking time: 0 minutes
Servings: 16

Ingredients:
- 8 eggs, hard-boiled, peeled, and mashed with a fork
- 4 ounces black caviar
- 4 ounces red caviar
- Salt and ground black pepper, to taste
- 1 onion, peeled and diced
- ¾ cup mayonnaise
- Toast baguette slices, for serving

Directions:
In a bowl, mix the mashed eggs with the mayonnaise, salt, pepper, and onion, and stir well. Spread the egg mixture on toasted baguette slices, and top each with caviar.

Nutrition: Calories - 122, Fat - 8, Fiber - 1, Carbs - 4, Protein - 7

Marinated Kebabs

Preparation time: 20 minutes
Cooking time: 10 minutes
Servings: 6

Ingredients:
- 1 red bell pepper, seeded, and cut into chunks
- 1 green bell pepper, seeded, and cut into chunks
- 1 orange bell pepper, seeded, and cut into chunks
- 2 pounds sirloin steak, cut into medium-sized cubes
- 4 garlic cloves, peeled and minced
- 1 onion, peeled and cut into chunks
- Salt and ground black pepper, to taste
- 2 tablespoons Dijon mustard
- 2, and ½ tablespoons Worcestershire sauce
- ¼ cup tamari sauce
- ¼ cup lemon juice
- ½ cup olive oil

Directions:
In a bowl, mix the Worcestershire sauce with salt, pepper, garlic, mustard, tamari, lemon juice, and oil, and whisk. Add the beef, bell peppers, and onion to this mixture, toss to coat, and set aside for a few minutes. Arrange the bell pepper, meat, and onion on skewers, alternating colors, place them on a preheated grill over medium-high heat, cook for 5 minutes on each side, transfer to a platter, and serve.

Nutrition: Calories - 246, Fat - 12, Fiber - 1, Carbs - 4, Protein - 26

Zucchini Rolls

Preparation time: 10 minutes
Cooking time: 5 minutes
Servings: 24

Ingredients:
- 2 tablespoons olive oil
- 3 zucchini, sliced thin
- 24 fresh basil leaves
- 2 tablespoons fresh mint, chopped
- 1⅓ cup ricotta cheese
- Salt and ground black pepper, to taste
- ¼ cup fresh basil, chopped
- Tomato sauce, for serving

Directions:
Brush the zucchini slices with the olive oil, season with salt and pepper on both sides, place them on preheated grill over medium heat, cook them for 2 minutes, flip, and cook for another 2 minutes. Place the zucchini slices on a plate, and set aside. In a bowl, mix the ricotta with the chopped basil, mint, salt, and pepper, and stir well. Spread this over the zucchini slices, divide the basil leaves as well, roll, and serve as an appetizer with some tomato sauce on the side.

Nutrition: Calories - 40, Fat - 3, Fiber - 0. 3, Carbs - 1, Protein - 2

Green Crackers

Preparation time: 10 minutes
Cooking time: 24 hours
Servings: 6

Ingredients:
- 2 cups flaxseeds, ground
- 2 cups flaxseeds, soaked overnight, and drained
- 4 bunches kale, chopped
- 1 bunch fresh basil, chopped
- ½ bunch celery, chopped
- 4 garlic cloves, peeled and minced
- ⅓ cup olive oil

Directions:
In a food processor, mix the ground flaxseed with celery, kale, basil, and garlic, and blend well. Add the oil, and soaked flaxseed, and blend again. Spread this on a tray, cut into medium crackers, introduce in a dehydrator, and dry for 24 hours at 115°F, turning them halfway. Arrange them on a platter and serve.

Nutrition: Calories - 100, Fat - 1, Fiber - 2, Carbs - 1, Protein - 4

Cheese and Pesto Terrine

Preparation time: 30 minutes
Cooking time: 0 minutes
Servings: 10

Ingredients:
- ½ cup heavy cream
- 10 ounces goat cheese, crumbled
- 3 tablespoons basil pesto
- Salt and ground black pepper, to taste
- 5 sundried tomatoes, cored and chopped
- ¼ cup pine nuts + and 1 tablespoon pine nuts, toasted and chopped

Directions:
In a bowl, mix the goat cheese with the heavy cream, salt, and pepper, and stir using a mixer. Spoon half of this mixture into a lined bowl and spread. Add the pesto on top and spread this as well. Add another layer of cheese, then add the sundried tomatoes and ¼ cup pine nuts. Spread one final layer of cheese, and top with 1 tablespoon pine nuts. Keep in the refrigerator for a couple of hours, turn upside down on a plate, and serve.

Nutrition: Calories - 240, Fat - 12, Fiber - 3, Carbs - 5, Protein - 12

Avocado Salsa

Preparation time: 10 minutes
Cooking time: 0 minutes
Servings: 4

Ingredients:
- 1 onion, peeled and chopped
- 2 avocados, pitted, peeled, and chopped
- 3 jalapeño pepper, chopped
- Salt and ground black pepper, to taste
- 2 tablespoons cumin powder
- 2 tablespoons lime juice
- ½ tomato, cored and chopped

Directions:
In a bowl, mix the onion with the avocado, peppers, salt, black pepper, cumin, lime juice, and tomato pieces, and stir well. Transfer this to a bowl and serve with toasted baguette slices.

Nutrition: Calories - 120, Fat - 2, Fiber - 2, Carbs - 0. 4, Protein - 4

Egg Chips

Preparation time: 5 minutes
Cooking time: 10 minutes
Servings: 2

Ingredients:
- ½ tablespoon water
- 2 tablespoons Parmesan cheese, shredded
- 4 eggs whites
- Salt and ground black pepper, to taste

Directions:
In a bowl, mix the egg whites with salt, pepper, and water, and whisk. Spoon this into a muffin pan, sprinkle cheese on top, place in an oven at 400°F, and bake for 15 minutes. Transfer the egg white chips to a platter and serve.

Nutrition: Calories - 120, Fat - 2, Fiber - 1, Carbs - 2, Protein - 7

Chili Lime Chips

Preparation time: 10 minutes
Cooking time: 20 minutes
Servings: 4

Ingredients:
- 1 cup almond flour
- Salt and ground black pepper, to taste
- 1½ teaspoons lime zest
- 1 teaspoon lime juice
- 1 egg

Directions:
In a bowl, mix the almond flour with lime zest, lime juice, and salt, and stir. Add the egg, and whisk again. Divide this into 4 parts, roll each into a ball, and then spread well using a rolling pin. Cut each into 6 triangles, place them all on a lined baking sheet, place in an oven at 350°F, and bake for 20 minutes.

Nutrition: Calories - 90, Fat - 1, Fiber - 1, Carbs - 0. 6, Protein - 3

Artichoke Dip

Preparation time: 10 minutes
Cooking time: 15 minutes
Servings: 16

Ingredients:
- ¼ cup sour cream
- ¼ cup heavy cream
- ¼ cup mayonnaise
- ¼ cup shallot, peeled and chopped
- 1 tablespoon olive oil
- 2 garlic cloves, peeled and minced
- 4 ounces cream cheese
- ½ cup Parmesan cheese, grated
- 1 cup mozzarella cheese, shredded
- 4 ounces feta cheese, crumbled
- 1 tablespoon balsamic vinegar
- 28 ounces canned artichoke hearts, chopped
- Salt and ground black pepper, to taste
- 10 ounces spinach, chopped

Directions:
Heat up a pan with the oil over medium heat, add the shallot and garlic, stir, and cook for 3 minutes. Add the heavy cream and cream cheese, and stir. Add sour cream, Parmesan cheese, mayonnaise, feta cheese, and mozzarella cheese, stir, and reduce heat. Add the artichoke, spinach, salt, pepper, and vinegar, stir well, take off the heat, transfer to a bowl, and serve.

Nutrition: Calories - 144, Fat - 12, Fiber - 2, Carbs - 5, Protein - 5

Ketogenic Fish and Seafood Recipes

Fish Pie

Preparation time: 10 minutes
Cooking time: 1 hour and 10 minutes
Servings: 6

Ingredients:
- 1 onion, peeled and chopped
- 2 salmon fillets, skinless and cut into medium-sized pieces
- 2 mackerel fillets, skinless and cut into medium-sized pieces
- 3 haddock fillets, cut into medium-sized pieces
- 2 bay leaves
- ¼ cup butter+ 2 tablespoons butter
- 1 cauliflower head, separated into florets
- 4 eggs
- 4 cloves
- 1 cup whipping cream
- ½ cup water
- A pinch of nutmeg, ground
- 1 teaspoon Dijon mustard
- 1 cup cheddar cheese, shredded+ ½ cup cheddar cheese, shredded
- Some chopped parsley
- Salt and ground black pepper, to taste
- 4 tablespoons fresh chives, chopped

Directions:
Put some water in a pan, add the some salt, bring to a boil over medium heat, add the eggs, cook them for 10 minutes, take off the heat, drain, leave them to cool down, peel, and cut them into quarters. Put the water in another pot, bring to a boil, add the cauliflower florets, cook for 10 minutes, drain them, transfer to a blender, add the ¼ cup butter, pulse well, and transfer to a bowl. Put the cream and ½ cup water in a pan, add the fish, toss to coat, and heat up over medium heat. Add the onion, cloves, and bay leaves, bring to a boil, reduce heat, and simmer for 10 minutes. Take off heat, transfer fish to a baking dish, and set aside. Return the pan with fish sauce to heat, add the nutmeg, stir, and cook for 5 minutes. Take off the heat, discard the cloves, and bay leaves, add the 1 cup cheddar cheese, and 2 tablespoons butter, and stir well. Place the egg quarters on top of the fish in the baking dish. Add the cream and cheese sauce over them, top with cauliflower mash, sprinkle the rest of the cheddar cheese, chives, and parsley, place in an oven at 400ºF for 30 minutes. Let the pie to cool before slicing, and serving.

Nutrition: Calories - 300, Fat - 45, Fiber - 3, Carbs - 5, Protein - 26

Baked Haddock

Preparation time: 10 minutes
Cooking time: 30 minutes
Servings: 4

Ingredients:
- 1 pound haddock
- 3 teaspoons water
- 2 tablespoons lemon juice
- Salt and ground black pepper, to taste
- 2 tablespoons mayonnaise
- 1 teaspoon dill weed
- Vegetable oil cooking spray
- A pinch of Old Bay Seasoning

Directions:
Spray a baking dish with some cooking oil. Add the lemon juice, water, and fish, and toss to coat a bit. Add the salt, pepper, Old Bay Seasoning, and dill, and toss again. Add the mayonnaise and spread well. Place in an oven at 350ºF, and bake for 30 minutes. Divide on plates and serve.

Nutrition: Calories - 104, Fat - 12, Fiber - 1, Carbs - 0. 5, Protein - 20

Tilapia

Preparation time: 10 minutes
Cooking time: 10 minutes
Servings: 4

Ingredients:
- 4 tilapia fillets, boneless
- Salt and ground black pepper, to taste
- ½ cup Parmesan cheese, grated
- 4 tablespoons mayonnaise
- ¼ teaspoon dried basil
- ¼ teaspoon garlic powder
- 2 tablespoons lemon juice
- ¼ cup butter
- Vegetable oil cooking spray
- A pinch of onion powder

Directions:
Spray a baking sheet with cooking spray, place tilapia on it, season with salt, and pepper, place under a preheated broiler, and cook for 3 minutes. Turn the fish and broil for 3 minutes. In a bowl, mix the Parmesan cheese with the mayonnaise, basil, garlic, lemon juice, onion powder, and butter, and stir well. Add the fish to this mixture, toss to coat well, place on baking sheet again, and broil for 3 minutes. Transfer to plates and serve.

Nutrition: Calories - 175, Fat - 10, Fiber - 0, Carbs - 2, Protein - 17

Trout with Special Sauce

Preparation time: 10 minutes
Cooking time: 10 minutes
Servings: 1

Ingredients:
- 1 trout fillet
- Salt and ground black pepper, to taste
- 1 tablespoon olive oil
- 1 tablespoon butter
- Zest, and juice from 1 orange
- ½ cup fresh parsley, chopped
- ½ cup pecans, chopped

Directions:
Heat up a pan with the oil over medium-high heat, add the fish fillet, season with salt, and pepper, cook for 4 minutes on each side, transfer to a plate, and keep warm. Heat up the same pan with the butter over medium heat, add the pecans, stir, and toast for 1 minutes. Add the orange juice, orange zest, some salt, and pepper, and chopped parsley, stir, cook for 1 minute, and pour over the fish fillets, and serve.

Nutrition: Calories - 200, Fat - 10, Fiber - 2, Carbs - 1, Protein - 14

Trout with Butter Sauce

Preparation time: 10 minutes
Cooking time: 10 minutes
Servings: 4

Ingredients:
- 4 trout fillets
- Salt and ground black pepper, to taste
- 3 teaspoons lemon zest, grated
- 3 tablespoons fresh chives, chopped
- 6 tablespoons butter
- 2 tablespoons olive oil
- 2 teaspoons lemon juice

Directions:
Season the trout with salt, and pepper, drizzle the olive oil, and massage a bit. Heat up a kitchen grill over medium-high heat, add the fish fillets, cook for 4 minutes, flip, and cook for 4 minutes. Heat up a pan with the butter over medium heat, add the salt, pepper, chives, lemon juice, and lemon zest, and stir well. Divide the fish fillets on plates, drizzle the butter sauce over them, and serve.

Nutrition: Calories - 320, Fat - 12, Fiber - 1, Carbs - 2, Protein - 24

Roasted Salmon

Preparation time: 10 minutes
Cooking time: 12 minutes
Servings: 4

Ingredients:
- 2 tablespoons butter, softened
- 1¼ pound salmon fillet
- 2 ounces kimchi, diced
- Salt and ground black pepper, to taste

Directions:
In a food processor, mix the butter with kimchi, and blend well. Rub the salmon with salt, pepper, and kimchi mixture, and place into a baking dish. Place in an oven at 425°F, and bake for 15 minutes. Divide on plates and serve.

Nutrition: Calories - 200, Fat - 12, Fiber - 0, Carbs - 3, Protein - 21

Salmon Meatballs

Preparation time: 10 minutes
Cooking time: 30 minutes
Servings: 4

Ingredients:
- 2 tablespoons butter
- 2 garlic cloves, peeled and minced
- ⅓ cup onion, peeled and chopped
- 1 pound wild salmon, boneless and minced
- ¼ cup fresh chives, chopped
- 1 egg
- 2 tablespoons Dijon mustard
- 1 tablespoon coconut flour
- Salt and ground black pepper, to taste

For the sauce:
- 4 garlic cloves, peeled and minced
- 2 tablespoons butter
- 2 tablespoons Dijon mustard
- Juice, and zest of 1 lemon
- 2 cups coconut cream
- 2 tablespoons fresh chives, chopped

Directions:
Heat up a pan with 2 tablespoons butter over medium heat, add the onion, and 2 garlic cloves, stir, cook for 3 minutes, and transfer to a bowl. In another bowl, mix the onion and garlic with the salmon, chives, coconut flour, salt, pepper, 2 tablespoons mustard, and egg, and stir well. Shape meatballs from the salmon mixture, place on a baking sheet, place in an oven at 350°F, and bake for 25 minutes. Heat up a pan with 2 tablespoons butter over medium heat, add the 4 garlic cloves, stir, and cook for 1 minute. Add the coconut cream, 2 tablespoons Dijon mustard, lemon juice, lemon zest, and chives, stir, and cook for 3 minutes. Take the salmon meatballs out of the oven, drop them into the Dijon sauce, toss, cook for 1 minute, and take off the heat. Divide into bowls and serve.

Nutrition: Calories - 171, Fat - 5, Fiber - 1, Carbs - 6, Protein - 23

Salmon with Caper Sauce

Preparation time: 10 minutes
Cooking time: 20 minutes
Servings: 3

Ingredients:
- 3 salmon fillets
- Salt and ground black pepper, to taste
- 1 tablespoon olive oil
- 1 tablespoon Italian seasoning
- 2 tablespoons capers
- 3 tablespoons lemon juice
- 4 garlic cloves, peeled and minced
- 2 tablespoons butter

Directions:
Heat up a pan with the olive oil over medium heat, add the fish fillets skin side up, season them with salt, pepper, and Italian seasoning, cook for 2 minutes, flip, and cook for 2 minutes, take off the heat, cover pan, and set aside for 15 minutes. Transfer the fish to a plate, and leave them aside. Heat up the same pan over medium heat, add the capers, lemon juice, and garlic, stir, and cook for 2 minutes. Take the pan off the heat, add the butter, and stir well. Return the fish to pan, and toss to coat with the sauce. Divide on plates and serve.

Nutrition: Calories - 245, Fat - 12, Fiber - 1, Carbs - 3, Protein - 23

Simple Grilled Oysters

Preparation time: 10 minutes
Cooking time: 10 minutes
Servings: 3

Ingredients:
- 6 oysters, shucked
- 3 garlic cloves, peeled and minced
- 1 lemon, cut in wedges
- 1 tablespoon parsley
- A pinch of sweet paprika
- 2 tablespoons melted butter

Directions:
Top each oyster with melted butter, parsley, paprika, and butter. Place them on preheated grill over medium-high heat, and cook for 8 minutes. Serve them with lemon wedges on the side.

Nutrition: Calories - 60, Fat - 1, Fiber - 0, Carbs - 0. 6, Protein - 1

Baked Halibut

Preparation time: 10 minutes
Cooking time: 10 minutes
Servings: 4

Ingredients:
- ½ cup Parmesan cheese, grated
- ¼ cup butter
- ¼ cup mayonnaise
- 2 tablespoons green onions, chopped
- 6 garlic cloves, peeled and minced
- A dash of Tabasco sauce
- 4 halibut fillets
- Salt and ground black pepper, to taste
- Juice of ½ lemon

Directions:
Season the halibut with salt, pepper, and some of the lemon juice, place in a baking dish, and cook in the oven at 450°F for 6 minutes. Heat up a pan with the butter over medium heat, add the Parmesan cheese, mayonnaise, green onions, Tabasco sauce, garlic, and the rest of the lemon juice, and stir well. Take the fish out of the oven, drizzle the cheese sauce all over, turn the oven to broil, and broil the fish for 3 minutes. Divide on plates and serve.

Nutrition: Calories - 240, Fat - 12, Fiber - 1, Carbs - 5, Protein - 23

Crusted Salmon

Preparation time: 10 minutes
Cooking time: 15 minutes
Servings: 4

Ingredients:
- 3 garlic cloves, peeled and minced
- 2 pounds salmon fillet
- Salt and ground black pepper, to taste
- ½ cup Parmesan cheese, grated
- ¼ cup fresh parsley, chopped

Directions:
Place the salmon on a lined baking sheet, season with salt, and pepper, cover with a parchment paper, place in an oven at 425°F, and bake for 10 minutes. Take the fish out of the oven, sprinkle Parmesan cheese, parsley, and garlic over fish, place in an oven again, and cook for 5 minutes. Divide on plates and serve.

Nutrition: Calories - 240, Fat - 12, Fiber - 1, Carbs - 0. 6, Protein - 25

Sour Cream Salmon

Preparation time: 10 minutes
Cooking time: 15 minutes
Servings: 4

Ingredients:
- 4 salmon fillets
- A drizzle of olive oil
- Salt and ground black pepper, to taste
- ⅓ cup Parmesan cheese, grated
- 1½ teaspoon mustard
- ½ cup sour cream

Directions:
Place the salmon on a lined baking sheet, season with salt, and pepper, and drizzle the oil. In a bowl, mix the sour cream with Parmesan cheese, mustard, salt, and pepper, and stir well. Spoon the sour cream mixture over the salmon, place in an oven at 350°F, and bake for 15 minutes. Divide on plates and serve.

Nutrition: Calories - 200, Fat - 6, Fiber - 1, Carbs - 4, Protein – 20

Grilled Salmon

Preparation time: 30 minutes
Cooking time: 10 minutes
Servings: 4

Ingredients:
- 4 salmon fillets
- 1 tablespoon olive oil
- Salt and ground black pepper, to taste
- 1 teaspoon cumin
- 1 teaspoon sweet paprika
- ½ teaspoon chili powder
- 1 teaspoon onion powder

For the salsa:
- 1 onion, peeled and chopped
- 1 avocado, pitted, peeled, and chopped
- 2 tablespoons fresh cilantro, chopped
- Juice from 2 limes
- Salt and ground black pepper, to taste

Directions:
In a bowl, mix the salt, pepper, chili powder, onion powder, paprika, and cumin. Rub the salmon with this mixture, drizzle the oil, and rub again, and cook on preheated grill for 4 minutes on each side. In a bowl, mix the avocado with the onion, salt, pepper, cilantro, and lime juice, and stir. Divide the salmon on plates, and top each fillet with avocado salsa.

Nutrition: Calories - 300, Fat - 14, Fiber - 4, Carbs - 5, Protein - 20

Tuna Cakes

Preparation time: 10 minutes
Cooking time: 10 minutes
Servings: 12

Ingredients:
- 15 ounces canned tuna, drained well and flaked
- 3 eggs
- ½ teaspoon dried dill
- 1 teaspoon dried parsley
- ½ cup onion chopped
- 1 teaspoon garlic powder
- Salt and ground black pepper, to taste
- Oil, for frying

Directions:
In a bowl, mix the tuna with salt, pepper, dill, parsley, onion, garlic powder, and eggs, and stir well. Shape the tuna cakes and place on a plate. Heat up a pan with some oil over medium-high heat, add the tuna cakes, cook for 5 minutes on each side. Divide on plates and serve.

Nutrition: Calories - 140, Fat - 2, Fiber - 1, Carbs - 0. 6, Protein - 6

Pan-roasted Cod

Preparation time: 10 minutes
Cooking time: 20 minutes
Servings: 4

Ingredients:
- 1 pound cod, cut into medium-sized pieces
- Salt and ground black pepper, to taste
- 2 green onions, chopped
- 3 garlic cloves, peeled and minced
- 3 tablespoons soy sauce
- 1 cup fish stock
- 1 tablespoons balsamic vinegar
- 1 tablespoon fresh ginger, grated
- ½ teaspoon red chili flakes

Directions:
Heat up a pan over medium-high heat, add the fish pieces, and brown them a few minutes on each side. Add the garlic, green onions, salt, pepper, soy sauce, fish stock, vinegar, chili pepper, and ginger, stir, cover, reduce heat, and cook for 20 minutes. Divide on plates and serve.

Nutrition: Calories - 154, Fat - 3, Fiber - 0. 5, Carbs - 4, Protein - 24

Sea Bass with Capers

Preparation time: 10 minutes
Cooking time: 15 minutes
Servings: 4

Ingredients:
- 1 lemon, sliced
- 1 pound sea bass fillet
- 2 tablespoons capers
- 2 tablespoons fresh dill
- Salt and ground black pepper, to taste

Directions:
Put the sea bass fillet into a baking dish, season with salt, and pepper, add the capers, dill, and lemon slices on top. Place in an oven at 350°F, and bake for 15 minutes. Divide on plates and serve.

Nutrition: Calories - 150, Fat - 3, Fiber - 2, Carbs - 0. 7, Protein - 5

Cod with Arugula

Preparation time: 10 minutes
Cooking time: 20 minutes
Servings: 2

Ingredients:
- 2 cod fillets
- 1 tablespoon olive oil
- Salt and ground black pepper, to taste
- Juice of 1 lemon
- 3 cup arugula
- ½ cup black olives, pitted and sliced
- 2 tablespoons capers
- 1 garlic clove, peeled and chopped

Directions:
Arrange the fish fillets in a heatproof dish, season with salt, pepper, drizzle the oil, and lemon juice, toss to coat, place in an oven at 450°F, and bake for 20 minutes. In a food processor, mix the arugula with salt, pepper, capers, olives, and garlic, and blend well. Arrange the fish on plates, top with arugula tapenade, and serve.

Nutrition: Calories - 240, Fat - 5, Fiber - 3, Carbs - 3, Protein - 10

Baked Halibut with Vegetables

Preparation time: 10 minutes
Cooking time: 35 minutes
Servings: 2

Ingredients:
- 1 red bell pepper, seeded and chopped
- 1 yellow bell pepper, seeded and chopped
- 1 teaspoon balsamic vinegar
- 1 tablespoon olive oil
- 2 halibut fillets
- 2 cups baby spinach
- Salt and ground black pepper, to taste
- 1 teaspoon cumin

Directions:
In a bowl, mix the bell peppers with salt, pepper, half of the oil, and the vinegar, toss to coat well, and transfer to a baking dish. Place in an oven at 400ºF, and bake for 20 minutes. Heat up a pan with the rest of the oil over medium heat, add the fish, season with salt, pepper, and cumin, and brown on all sides. Take the baking dish out of the oven, add the spinach, stir gently, and divide the whole mixture on plates. Add the fish on the side, sprinkle with salt and pepper, and serve.

Nutrition: Calories - 230, Fat - 12, Fiber - 1, Carbs - 4, Protein - 9

Fish Curry

Preparation time: 10 minutes
Cooking time: 25 minutes
Servings: 4

Ingredients:
- 4 white fish fillets
- ½ teaspoon mustard seeds
- Salt and ground black pepper, to taste
- 2 green chilies, chopped
- 1 teaspoon fresh ginger, grated
- 1 teaspoon curry powder
- ¼ teaspoon cumin
- 4 tablespoons coconut oil
- 1 onion, peeled and chopped
- 1-inch turmeric root, grated
- ¼ cup fresh cilantro
- 1½ cups coconut cream
- 3 garlic cloves, peeled and minced

Directions:
Heat up a pot with half of the coconut oil over medium heat, add the mustard seeds, and cook for 2 minutes. Add the ginger, onion, and garlic, stir, and cook for 5 minutes. Add the turmeric, curry powder, chilies, and cumin, stir, and cook for 5 minutes. Add the coconut milk, salt, and pepper, stir, bring to a boil, and cook for 15 minutes. Heat up another pan with the rest of the oil over medium heat, add the fish, stir, and cook for 3 minutes. Add this to the curry sauce, stir, and cook for 5 minutes. Add the cilantro, stir, divide into bowls, and serve.

Nutrition: Calories - 500, Fat - 34, Fiber - 7, Carbs - 6, Protein - 44

Sautéed Lemon Shrimp

Preparation time: 10 minutes
Cooking time: 10 minutes
Servings: 4

Ingredients:
- 2 tablespoons olive oil
- 1 tablespoon butter
- 1 pound shrimp, peeled and deveined
- 2 tablespoons lemon juice
- 2 tablespoons garlic, minced
- 1 tablespoon lemon zest
- Salt and ground black pepper, to taste

Directions:
Heat up a pan with the oil and butter over medium-high heat, add the shrimp, and cook for 2 minutes. Add the garlic, stir, and cook for 4 minutes. Add the lemon juice, lemon zest, salt, and pepper, stir, take off the heat, and serve.

Nutrition: Calories - 149, Fat - 1, Fiber - 3, Carbs - 1, Protein - 6

Roasted Sea Bass

Preparation time: 10 minutes
Cooking time: 12 minutes
Servings: 4

Ingredients:
- 2 sea bass fillets
- 2 teaspoon olive oil
- 2 teaspoons Italian seasoning
- ¼ cup green olives, pitted and chopped
- ¼ cup cherry tomatoes, cored and chopped
- ¼ cup black olives, chopped
- 1 tablespoon lemon zest
- 2 tablespoons lemon zest
- Salt and ground black pepper, to taste
- 2 tablespoons fresh parsley, chopped
- 1 tablespoon olive oil

Directions:
Rub the fish with salt, pepper, Italian seasoning, and 2 teaspoons olive oil, transfer to a baking dish, and set aside. In a bowl, mix the tomatoes with all the olives, salt, pepper, lemon zest, and lemon juice, parsley, and 1 tablespoon olive oil, and toss well. Place the fish in the oven at 400°F, and bake for 12 minutes. Divide the fish on plates, top with tomato relish, and serve.

Nutrition: Calories - 150, Fat - 4, Fiber - 2, Carbs - 1, Protein - 10

Coconut Shrimp

Preparation time: 10 minutes
Cooking time: 13 minutes
Servings: 4

Ingredients:
- 1 pound shrimp, peeled and deveined
- Salt and ground black pepper, to taste
- 4 cherry tomatoes, cored and chopped
- 2 cups sugar snap peas, sliced lengthwise
- 1 red bell pepper, seeded and sliced
- 1 tablespoon olive oil
- ½ cup fresh cilantro, chopped
- 1 tablespoon garlic, minced
- ½ cup green onion, peeled and chopped
- ½ teaspoon red pepper flakes
- 10 ounces coconut milk
- 2 tablespoons lime juice

Directions:
Heat up a pan with the oil over medium-high heat, add the snap peas, and stir-fry for 2 minutes. Add the pepper, and cook for 3 minutes. Add the cilantro, garlic, green onions, and pepper flakes, stir, and cook for 1 minute. Add the tomatoes, and coconut milk, stir, and simmer everything for 5 minutes. Add the shrimp and lime juice, stir, and cook for 3 minutes. Season with salt and pepper, stir, and serve hot.

Nutrition: Calories - 150, Fat - 3, Fiber - 3, Carbs - 1, Protein - 7

Shrimp and Noodle Salad

Preparation time: 10 minutes
Cooking time: 0 minutes
Servings: 4

Ingredients:
- 1 cucumber, cut with a spiralizer
- ½ cup fresh basil, chopped
- ½ pound shrimp, already cooked, peeled and deveined
- Salt and ground black pepper, to taste
- 1 tablespoon stevia
- 2 teaspoons fish sauce
- 2 tablespoons lime juice
- 2 teaspoons chili garlic sauce

Directions:
Put the cucumber noodles on a paper towel, cover with another one, and press well. Put into a bowl and mix with basil, shrimp, salt, and pepper. In another bowl, mix the stevia with fish sauce, lime juice, and chili sauce, and whisk. Add this to the shrimp salad, toss to coat well, and serve.

Nutrition: Calories - 130, Fat - 2, Fiber - 3, Carbs - 1, Protein - 6

Roasted Mahi Mahi and Salsa

Preparation time: 10 minutes
Cooking time: 16 minutes
Servings: 2

Ingredients:
- 2 mahi mahi fillets
- ½ cup onion, peeled and chopped
- 4 teaspoons olive oil
- 1 teaspoon Greek seasoning
- 1 teaspoon garlic, minced
- 1 green bell pepper, seeded and chopped
- ½ cup canned tomato salsa
- 2 tablespoons Kalamata olives, pitted and chopped
- ¼ cup chicken stock
- Salt and ground black pepper, to taste
- 2 tablespoons feta cheese, crumbled

Directions:
Heat up a pan with 2 teaspoons oil over medium heat, add the bell pepper and onion, stir, and cook for 3 minutes. Add the Greek seasoning and garlic, stir, and cook for 1 minute. Add the stock, olives, and salsa, stir again, and cook for 5 minutes or until the mixture thickens. Transfer to a bowl and set aside. Heat up the pan again with the rest of the oil over medium heat, add the fish, season with salt and pepper, and cook for 2 minutes. Flip, cook for 2 minutes, and transfer to a baking dish. Spoon the salsa over fish, place in an oven, and bake at 425°F for 6 minutes. Sprinkle feta on top and serve hot.

Nutrition: Calories - 200, Fat - 5, Fiber - 2, Carbs - 2, Protein - 7

Spicy Shrimp

Preparation time: 10 minutes
Cooking time: 8 minutes
Servings: 2

Ingredients:
- ½ pound shrimp, peeled and deveined
- 2 teaspoons Worcestershire sauce
- 2 teaspoons olive oil
- Juice of 1 lemon
- Salt and ground black pepper, to taste
- 1 teaspoon Creole seasoning

Directions:
Arrange the shrimp in one layer in a baking dish, season with salt, and pepper, and drizzle the oil. Add the Worcestershire sauce, lemon juice, and sprinkle Creole seasoning. Toss the shrimp in the seasoning, place in an oven, set it under the broiler, and broil for 8 minutes. Divide between 2 plates and serve.

Nutrition: Calories - 120, Fat - 3, Fiber - 1, Carbs - 2, Protein - 6

Shrimp Stew

Preparation time: 10 minutes
Cooking time: 15 minutes
Servings: 6

Ingredients:
- ¼ cup onion, peeled and chopped
- ¼ cup olive oil
- 1 garlic clove, peeled and minced
- 1½ pounds shrimp, peeled and deveined
- ¼ cup red pepper, roasted and chopped
- 14 ounces canned diced tomatoes
- ¼ cup fresh cilantro, chopped
- 2 tablespoons sriracha sauce
- 1 cup coconut milk
- Salt and ground black pepper, to taste
- 2 tablespoons lime juice

Directions:
Heat up a pan with the oil over medium heat, add the onion, stir, and cook for 4 minutes. Add the peppers and garlic, stir, and cook for 4 minutes. Add the cilantro, tomatoes, and shrimp, stir, and cook until shrimp turn pink. Add the coconut milk and sriracha sauce, stir, and bring to a gentle simmer. Add the salt, pepper, and lime juice, stir, transfer to bowls, and serve.

Nutrition: Calories - 250, Fat - 12, Fiber - 3, Carbs - 5, Protein - 20

Shrimp Alfredo

Preparation time: 10 minutes
Cooking time: 20 minutes
Servings: 4

Ingredients:
- 8 ounces mushrooms, chopped
- 1 asparagus bunch, cut into medium-sized pieces
- 1 pound shrimp, peeled and deveined
- Salt and ground black pepper, to taste
- 1 spaghetti squash, cut in half
- 2 tablespoons olive oil
- 2 teaspoons Italian seasoning
- 1 onion, peeled and chopped
- 1 teaspoon red pepper flakes
- ¼ cup butter
- 1 cup Parmesan cheese, grated
- 2 garlic cloves, peeled and minced
- 1 cup heavy cream

Directions:
Place the squash halves on a lined baking sheet, place in an oven at 425°F, and roast for 40 minutes. Scoop out the insides and put them into a bowl. Put water in a pot, add the some salt, bring to a boil over medium heat, add the asparagus, steam for a couple of minutes, transfer to a bowl filled with ice water, drain, and set aside as well. Heat up a pan with the oil over medium heat, add the onions and mushrooms, stir, and cook for 7 minutes. Add the pepper flakes, Italian seasoning, salt, pepper, squash, and asparagus, stir, and cook for a few minutes. Heat up another pan with the butter over medium heat, add the heavy cream, garlic, and Parmesan cheese, stir, and cook for 5 minutes. Add the shrimp to the pan, stir, and cook for 7 minutes. Divide the vegetables on plates, top with shrimp and sauce, and serve.

Nutrition: Calories - 455, Fat - 6, Fiber - 5, Carbs - 4, Protein - 13

Shrimp and Snow Pea Soup

Preparation time: 10 minutes
Cooking time: 10 minutes
Servings: 4

Ingredients:
- 4 scallions, chopped
- 1½ tablespoons coconut oil
- 1 small ginger root, diced
- 8 cups chicken stock
- ¼ cup coconut aminos
- 5 ounces canned bamboo shoots, drained and sliced
- Ground black pepper, to taste
- ¼ teaspoon fish sauce
- 1 pound shrimp, peeled and deveined
- ½ pound snow peas
- 1 tablespoon sesame oil
- ½ tablespoon chili oil

Directions:
Heat up a pot with the coconut oil over medium heat, add the scallions and ginger, stir, and cook for 2 minutes. Add the coconut aminos, stock, black pepper, and fish sauce, stir, and bring to a boil. Add the shrimp, snow peas, and bamboo shoots, stir, and cook for 3 minutes. Add the sesame oil and hot chili oil, stir, divide into bowls, and serve.

Nutrition: Calories - 200, Fat - 3, Fiber - 2, Carbs - 4, Protein - 14

Garlicky Mussels

Preparation time: 5 minutes
Cooking time: 5 minutes
Servings: 4

Ingredients:
- 2 pound mussels, debearded and scrubbed
- 2 garlic cloves, peeled and minced
- 1 tablespoon butter
- A splash of lemon juice

Directions:
Put some water in a pot, add the mussels, bring to a boil over medium heat, cook for 5 minutes, take off the heat, discard any unopened mussels, and transfer them to a bowl. In another bowl, mix the butter with garlic and lemon juice, whisk, and heat up in the microwave for 1 minute. Pour over mussels and serve.

Nutrition: Calories - 50, Fat - 1, Fiber - 0, Carbs - 0. 5, Protein - 2

Fried Calamari with Spicy Sauce

Preparation time: 10 minutes
Cooking time: 20 minutes
Servings: 2

Ingredients:
- 1 squid, cut into medium rings
- A pinch of cayenne pepper
- 1 egg, whisked
- 2 tablespoons coconut flour
- Salt and ground black pepper, to taste
- Coconut oil for frying
- 1 tablespoons lemon juice
- 4 tablespoons mayonnaise
- 1 teaspoon sriracha sauce

Directions:
Season the squid rings with salt, pepper, and cayenne pepper, and put them in a bowl. In another bowl, mix the egg with salt, pepper, and coconut flour, and whisk. Dredge the calamari rings in the egg mixture. Heat up a pan with enough coconut oil over medium heat, add the calamari rings, cook them until they become golden brown on both sides. Transfer to paper towels, drain the excess grease, and put in a bowl. In another bowl, mix the mayonnaise with the lemon juice and sriracha sauce, stir well, and serve the calamari rings with this sauce on the side.

Nutrition: Calories - 345, Fat - 32, Fiber - 3, Carbs - 3, Protein - 13

Baked Calamari and Shrimp

Preparation time: 10 minutes
Cooking time: 20 minutes
Servings: 1

Ingredients:
- 8 ounces calamari, cut into medium rings
- 7 ounces shrimp, peeled and deveined
- 1 eggs
- 3 tablespoons coconut flour
- 1 tablespoon coconut oil
- 2 tablespoons avocado, chopped
- 1 teaspoon tomato paste
- 1 tablespoon mayonnaise
- A splash of Worcestershire sauce
- 1 teaspoon lemon juice
- 2 lemon slices
- Salt and ground black pepper, to taste
- ½ teaspoon turmeric

Directions:
In a bowl, whisk the egg with the coconut oil. Add the calamari rings and shrimp, and toss to coat. In another bowl, mix the flour with salt, pepper, and turmeric and stir. Dredge the calamari and shrimp in this mixture, place everything on a lined baking sheet, place in an oven at 400ºF, and bake for 10 minutes. Flip the calamari and shrimp, and bake for 10 minutes. In a bowl, mix the avocado with the mayonnaise and tomato paste, and mash using a fork. Add the Worcestershire sauce, lemon juice, salt, and pepper, and stir well. Divide the calamari and shrimp on plates and serve with the sauce and lemon slices on the side.

Nutrition: Calories - 368, Fat - 23, Fiber - 3, Carbs - 10, Protein - 34

Octopus Salad

Preparation time: 10 minutes
Cooking time: 40 minutes
Servings: 2

Ingredients:
- 21 ounces octopus, rinsed
- Juice of 1 lemon
- 4 celery stalks, chopped
- 3 ounces olive oil
- Salt and ground black pepper, to taste
- 4 tablespoons fresh parsley, chopped

Directions:
Put the octopus in a pot, add enough water to cover them, cover the pot, bring to a boil over medium heat, cook for 40 minutes, drain, and set aside to cool down. Chop the octopus and put it in a salad bowl. Add the celery stalks, parsley, oil, and lemon juice, and toss well. Season with salt and pepper, toss again, and serve.

Nutrition: Calories - 140, Fat - 10, Fiber - 3, Carbs - 6, Protein - 23

Clam Chowder

Preparation time: 10 minutes
Cooking time: 2 hours
Servings: 4

Ingredients:
- 1 cup celery stalks, chopped
- Salt and ground black pepper, to taste
- 1 teaspoon ground thyme
- 2 cups chicken stock
- 14 ounces canned baby clams
- 2 cups heavy cream
- 1 cup onion, peeled and chopped
- 12 bacon slices, chopped

Directions:
Heat up a pan over medium heat, add the bacon slices, brown them, transfer the bacon to a bowl, reserving the bacon grease in the pan. Heat up the pan again, add the celery and onion, stir, and cook for 5 minutes. Transfer everything, including the bacon, to a slow cooker with the baby clams, salt, pepper, stock, thyme, and cream, stir, and cook on high for 2 hours. Divide into bowls and serve.

Nutrition: Calories - 420, Fat - 22, Fiber - 0, Carbs - 5, Protein - 25

Flounder and Shrimp

Preparation time: 10 minutes
Cooking time: 20 minutes
Servings: 4

Ingredients:
For the seasoning:
- 2 teaspoons onion powder
- 2 teaspoons dried thyme
- 2 teaspoons sweet paprika
- 2 teaspoons garlic powder
- Salt and ground black pepper, to taste
- ½ teaspoon allspice
- 1 teaspoon dried oregano
- A pinch of cayenne pepper
- ¼ teaspoon ground nutmeg
- ¼ teaspoon ground cloves
- A pinch of ground cinnamon

For the etouffee:
- 2 shallots, peeled and chopped
- 1 tablespoon butter
- 8 ounces bacon, sliced
- 1 green bell pepper, seeded and chopped
- 1 celery stalk, chopped
- 2 tablespoons coconut flour
- 1 tomato, cored and chopped
- 4 garlic cloves, peeled and minced
- 8 ounces shrimp, peeled, deveined, and chopped
- 2 cups chicken stock
- 1 tablespoon coconut milk
- ½ cup fresh parsley, chopped
- 1 teaspoon Tabasco sauce
- Salt and ground black pepper, to taste

For the flounder:
- 4 flounder fillets
- 2 tablespoons butter

Directions:
In a bowl, mix the paprika with thyme, garlic powder, onion powder, salt, pepper, oregano, allspice, cayenne pepper, cloves, nutmeg, and cinnamon, and stir. Reserve 2 tablespoons of this mixture, rub the flounder with the rest, and set aside. Heat up a pan over medium heat, add the bacon, stir, and cook for 6 minutes. Add the celery, bell pepper, shallots, and 1 tablespoon butter, stir, and cook for 4 minutes. Add the tomato and garlic, stir, and cook for 4 minutes. Add the coconut flour and reserved seasoning, stir, and cook for 2 minutes. Add the chicken stock and bring to a simmer. Heat up another pan with 2 tablespoons butter over medium-high heat, add the fish, cook for 2 minutes, flip, and cook for 2 minutes. Add the shrimp to the pan with the stock, stir, and cook for 2 minutes. Add the parsley, salt, pepper, coconut milk, and Tabasco sauce, stir, and take off the heat. Divide fish on plates, top with the shrimp sauce, and serve.

Nutrition: Calories - 200, Fat - 5, Fiber - 7, Carbs - 4, Protein - 20

Shrimp Salad

Preparation time: 10 minutes
Cooking time: 10 minutes
Servings: 4

Ingredients:
- 2 tablespoons olive oil
- 1 pound shrimp, peeled and deveined
- Salt and ground black pepper, to taste
- 2 tablespoons lime juice
- 3 endives, leaves separated
- 3 tablespoons fresh parsley, chopped
- 2 teaspoons fresh mint, chopped
- 1 tablespoon fresh tarragon, chopped
- 1 tablespoon lemon juice
- 2 tablespoons mayonnaise
- 1 teaspoon lime zest
- ½ cup sour cream

Directions:
In a bowl, mix the shrimp with salt, pepper, and olive oil, toss to coat, and spread them on a lined baking sheet. Place the shrimp in the oven at 400°F, and bake for 10 minutes. Add the shrimp to a bowl with the lime juice, toss them to coat, and set aside. In a bowl, mix the mayonnaise with sour cream, lime zest, lemon juice, salt, pepper, tarragon, mint, and parsley, and stir well. Chop shrimp, add this to salad dressing, toss to coat everything, spoon into the endive leaves, and serve.

Nutrition: Calories - 200, Fat - 11, Fiber - 2, Carbs - 1, Protein - 13

Fiery Oysters

Preparation time: 10 minutes
Cooking time: 0 minutes
Servings: 4

Ingredients:
- 12 oysters, shucked
- Juice of 1 lemon
- Juice from 1 orange
- Zest from 1 orange
- Juice from 1 lime
- Zest from 1 lime
- 2 tablespoons ketchup
- 1 Serrano chili pepper, chopped
- 1 cup tomato juice
- ½ teaspoon fresh ginger, grated
- ¼ teaspoon garlic, minced
- Salt, to taste
- ¼ cup olive oil
- ¼ cup fresh cilantro, chopped
- ¼ cup scallions, chopped

Directions:
In a bowl, mix the lemon juice, orange juice, orange zest, lime juice, lime zest, ketchup, chili pepper, tomato juice, ginger, garlic, oil, scallions, cilantro, and salt, and stir well. Spoon this onto oysters and serve them.

Nutrition: Calories - 100, Fat - 1, Fiber - 0, Carbs - 2, Protein - 5

Salmon Rolls

Preparation time: 10 minutes
Cooking time: 0 minutes
Servings: 12

Ingredients:
- 2 nori sheets
- 1 small avocado, pitted, peeled, and diced
- 6 ounces smoked salmon, sliced
- 4 ounces cream cheese
- 1 cucumber, sliced
- 1 teaspoon wasabi paste
- Picked ginger, for serving

Directions:
Place the nori sheets on a sushi mat. Divide salmon slices avocado, and cucumber slices on them. In a bowl, mix the cream cheese with the wasabi paste and stir well. Spread this over cucumber slices, roll the nori sheets, press well, cut each into 6 pieces, and serve with pickled ginger.

Nutrition: Calories - 80, Fat - 6, Fiber - 1, Carbs - 2, Protein - 4

Salmon Skewers

Preparation time: 10 minutes
Cooking time: 8 minutes
Servings: 4

Ingredients:
- 12 ounces salmon fillet, cubed
- 1 onion, peeled and cut into chunks
- ½ red bell pepper, seeded and cut in chunks
- ½ green bell pepper, seeded and cut in chunks
- ½ orange bell pepper, seeded and cut in chunks
- Juice from 1 lemon
- Salt and ground black pepper, to taste
- A drizzle of olive oil

Directions:
Thread skewers with the onion, bell peppers, and salmon cubes. Season them with salt and pepper, drizzle them with oil and lemon juice, and place them on preheated grill over medium-high heat. Cook for 4 minutes on each side, divide on plates, and serve.

Nutrition: Calories - 150, Fat - 3, Fiber - 6, Carbs - 3, Protein - 8

Grilled Shrimp

Preparation time: 20 minutes
Cooking time: 10 minutes
Servings: 4

Ingredients:
- 1 pound shrimp, peeled and deveined
- 1 tablespoon lemon juice
- 1 garlic clove, peeled and minced
- ½ cup fresh basil leaves
- 1 tablespoon pine nuts, toasted
- 2 tablespoons Parmesan cheese, grated
- 2 tablespoons olive oil
- Salt and ground black pepper, to taste

Directions:
In a food processor, mix the Parmesan cheese with the basil, garlic, pine nuts, oil, salt, pepper, and lemon juice, and blend well. Transfer this to a bowl, add the shrimp, toss to coat, and set aside for 20 minutes. Thread skewers with the marinated shrimp, place them on preheated grill over medium-high heat, cook for 3 minutes, flip, and cook for 3 minutes. Arrange on plates and serve.

Nutrition: Calories - 185, Fat - 11, Fiber - 0, Carbs - 2, Protein - 13

Calamari Salad

Preparation time: 30 minutes
Cooking time: 4 minutes
Servings: 4

Ingredients:
- 2 long red chilies, chopped
- 2 small red chilies, chopped
- 2 garlic cloves, peeled and minced
- 3 green onions, chopped
- 1 tablespoon balsamic vinegar
- Salt and ground black pepper, to taste
- Juice of 1 lemon
- 6 pounds calamari hoods, tentacles set aside
- 3. 5 ounces olive oil
- 3 ounces arugula, for serving

Directions:
In a bowl, mix the red chilies, green onions, vinegar, garlic, salt, pepper, lemon juice, and half of the oil, and stir well. Place the calamari and tentacles in a bowl, season with salt, and pepper, drizzle the rest of the oil, toss to coat, and place on preheated grill over medium-high heat. Cook for 2 minutes on each side, and transfer to the chili marinade. Toss to coat, and set aside for 30 minutes. Arrange the arugula on plates, top with the calamari and its marinade, and serve.

Nutrition: Calories - 200, Fat - 4, Fiber - 2, Carbs - 2, Protein - 7

Cod Salad

Preparation time: 2 hours and 10 minutes
Cooking time: 20 minutes
Servings: 8

Ingredients:
- 2 cups jarred pimiento peppers, chopped
- 2 pounds salt cod
- 1 cup fresh parsley, chopped
- 1 cup Kalamata olives, pitted and chopped
- 6 tablespoons capers
- ¾ cup olive oil
- Salt and ground black pepper, to taste
- Juice from 2 lemons
- 4 garlic cloves, peeled and minced
- 2 celery stalks, chopped
- ½ teaspoon red chili flakes
- 1 escarole head, leaves separated

Directions:
Put the cod in a pot, add the water to cover, bring to a boil over medium heat, boil for 20 minutes, drain, and cut into medium chunks. Put the cod in a salad bowl, add the peppers, parsley, olives, capers, celery, garlic, lemon juice, salt, pepper, olive oil, and chili flakes, and toss to coat. Arrange the escarole leaves on a platter, add cod salad, and serve.

Nutrition: Calories - 240, Fat - 4, Fiber - 2, Carbs - 6, Protein - 9

Sardine Salad

Preparation time: 10 minutes
Cooking time: 0 minutes
Servings: 1

Ingredients:
- 5 ounces canned sardines in oil
- 1 tablespoons lemon juice
- 1 small cucumber, chopped
- ½ tablespoon mustard
- Salt and ground black pepper, to taste

Directions:
Drain the sardines, put them in a bowl, and mash them using a fork. Add the salt, pepper, cucumber, lemon juice, and mustard, stir well, and serve cold.

Nutrition: Calories - 200, Fat - 20, Fiber - 1, Carbs - 0, Protein - 20

Italian Clams Delight

Preparation time: 10 minutes
Cooking time: 10 minutes
Servings: 6

Ingredients:
- ½ cup butter
- 36 clams, scrubbed
- 1 teaspoon red pepper flakes
- 1 teaspoon fresh parsley, chopped
- 5 garlic cloves, peeled and minced
- 1 tablespoon dried oregano
- 2 cups white wine

Directions:
Heat up a pan with the butter over medium heat, add the garlic, stir, and cook for 1 minute. Add the parsley, oregano, wine, and pepper flakes, and stir well. Add the clams, stir, cover, and cook for 10 minutes. Discard any unopened clams, ladle the clam mixture into bowls, and serve.

Nutrition: Calories - 224, Fat - 15, Fiber - 2, Carbs - 3, Protein - 4

Orange-glazed Salmon

Preparation time: 10 minutes
Cooking time: 10 minutes
Servings: 2

Ingredients:
- 2 lemons, sliced
- 1 pound wild salmon, skinless and cubed
- ¼ cup balsamic vinegar
- ¼ cup orange juice
- 1 teaspoon coconut oil
- ⅓ cup no-sugar added orange marmalade

Directions:
Heat up a pot over medium heat, add the vinegar, orange juice, and marmalade, stir well, bring to a simmer for 1 minute, reduce temperature, cook until it thickens a bit, and take off the heat. Arrange the salmon, and lemon slices on skewers, and brush them on one side with the orange glaze. Brush a kitchen grill with coconut oil and heat up over medium heat. Place salmon kebabs on grill with glazed side down, and cook for 4 minutes. Flip the kebabs, brush them with the rest of the orange glaze, cook for 4 minutes, and serve.

Nutrition: Calories - 160, Fat - 3, Fiber - 2, Carbs - 1, Protein - 8

Tuna and Chimichurri Sauce

Preparation time: 10 minutes
Cooking time: 5 minutes
Servings: 4

Ingredients:
- ½ cup fresh cilantro, chopped
- ⅓ cup olive oil
- 2 tablespoons olive oil
- 1 onion, peeled and chopped
- 3 tablespoon balsamic vinegar
- 2 tablespoons fresh parsley, chopped
- 2 tablespoons fresh basil, chopped
- 1 jalapeño pepper, chopped
- 1 pound sushi-grade tuna steak
- Salt and ground black pepper, to taste
- 1 teaspoon red pepper flakes
- 1 teaspoon fresh thyme, chopped
- A pinch of cayenne pepper
- 3 garlic cloves, peeled and minced
- 2 avocados, pitted, peeled, and sliced
- 6 ounces baby arugula

Directions:
In a bowl, mix the ⅓ cup oil with jalapeño, vinegar, onion, cilantro, basil, garlic, parsley, pepper flakes, thyme, cayenne, salt, and pepper, whisk, and set aside. Heat up a pan with the rest of the oil over medium-high heat, add the tuna, season with salt, and pepper, cook for 2 minutes on each side, transfer to a cutting board, set aside to cool, and slice. Mix the arugula with half of the chimichurri mixture and toss to coat. Divide the arugula on plates, top with tuna slices, drizzle the rest of the chimichurri sauce, and serve with avocado slices on the side.

Nutrition: Calories - 186, Fat - 3, Fiber - 1, Carbs - 4, Protein - 20

Salmon Bites with Chili Sauce

Preparation time: 10 minutes
Cooking time: 15 minutes
Servings: 6

Ingredients:
- 1¼ cups coconut, desiccated, and unsweetened
- 1 pound salmon, skinless and cubed
- 1 egg
- Salt and ground black pepper, to taste
- 1 tablespoon water
- ⅓ cup coconut flour
- 3 tablespoons coconut oil

For the sauce:
- ¼ teaspoon agar
- 3 garlic cloves, peeled and chopped
- ¾ cup water
- 4 red chili peppers, chopped
- ¼ cup balsamic vinegar
- ½ cup stevia
- A pinch of salt

Directions:
In a bowl, mix the flour with salt, and pepper, and stir. In another bowl, whisk the egg and 1 tablespoon water. Put the coconut in a third bowl. Dip the salmon cubes in flour, then in egg, and finally in coconut, and place them on a plate. Heat up a pan with the coconut oil over medium-high heat, add the salmon bites, cook for 3 minutes on each side, and transfer them to paper towels. Heat up a pan with ¾ cup water over high heat, sprinkle with the agar, and bring to a boil. Cook for 3 minutes, and take off the heat. In a blender, mix the garlic with the chilies, vinegar, stevia, and a pinch of salt, and blend well. Transfer this to a small pan, and heat up over medium-high heat. Stir, add the agar mixture, and cook for 3 minutes. Serve the salmon bites with chili sauce on the side.

Nutrition: Calories - 50, Fat - 2, Fiber - 0, Carbs - 4, Protein - 2

Irish Clams

Preparation time: 10 minutes
Cooking time: 10 minutes
Servings: 4

Ingredients:
- 2 pounds clams, scrubbed
- 3 ounces pancetta
- 1 tablespoon olive oil
- 3 tablespoons butter
- 2 garlic cloves, peeled and minced
- 1 bottle infused cider
- Salt and ground black pepper, to taste
- Juice of ½ lemon
- 1 green apple, cored and chopped
- 2 thyme sprigs, chopped

Directions:
Heat up a pan with the oil over medium-high heat, add the pancetta, brown for 3 minutes, and reduce temperature to medium. Add the butter, garlic, salt, pepper, and shallot, stir, and cook for 3 minutes. Increase the heat again, add the cider, stir well, and cook for 1 minute. Add the clams and thyme, cover pan, and simmer for 5 minutes. Discard any unopened clams, add the lemon juice and apple pieces, stir, and divide into bowls. Serve hot.

Nutrition: Calories - 100, Fat - 2, Fiber - 1, Carbs - 1, Protein - 20

Seared Scallops with Walnuts and Grapes

Preparation time: 5 minutes
Cooking time: 10 minutes
Servings: 4

Ingredients:
- 1 pound scallops
- 3 tablespoons olive oil
- 1 shallot, peeled and chopped
- 3 garlic cloves, peeled and minced
- 2 cups spinach
- 1 cup chicken stock
- 1½ cups red grapes, cut into halves
- ¼ cup walnuts, toasted and chopped
- 1 tablespoon butter
- Salt and ground black pepper, to taste

Directions:
Put the romanesco in a food processor, blend, and transfer to a bowl. Heat up a pan with 2 tablespoons oil over medium-high heat, add the shallot and garlic, stir, and cook for 1 minute. Add the romanesco, spinach, and 1 cup stock, stir, cook for 3 minutes, blend using an immersion blender, and take off the heat. Heat up another pan with 1 tablespoon oil, and the butter over medium-high heat, add the scallops, season with salt and pepper, cook for 2 minutes, flip, and sear for 1 minute. Divide romanesco mixture on plates, add the scallops on the side, top with walnuts and grapes, and serve.

Nutrition: Calories - 300, Fat - 12, Fiber - 2, Carbs - 6, Protein - 20

Oysters with Pico De Gallo

Preparation time: 10 minutes
Cooking time: 10 minutes
Servings: 6

Ingredients:
- 18 oysters, scrubbed
- ½ cup fresh cilantro, chopped
- 2 tomatoes, cored and chopped
- 1 jalapeño pepper, chopped
- ¼ cup onion, diced
- Salt and ground black pepper, to taste
- ½ cup Monterey Jack cheese, shredded
- 2 limes, cut into wedges
- Juice from 1 lime

Directions:
In a bowl, mix the onion with jalapeño, cilantro, tomatoes, salt, pepper, and lime juice, and stir well. Place the oysters on a preheated grill over medium-high heat, cover grill, and cook for 7 minutes until they open. Transfer the oysters to a heatproof dish, discarding any unopened ones. Top the oysters with cheese, and place under a preheated broiler for 1 minute. Arrange the oysters on a platter, top each with tomatoes mixture, and serve with lime wedges.

Nutrition: Calories - 70, Fat - 2, Fiber - 0, Carbs - 1, Protein - 1

Grilled Squid with Guacamole

Preparation time: 10 minutes
Cooking time: 10 minutes
Servings: 2

Ingredients:

- 2 medium squids, tentacles separated and tubes scored lengthwise
- A drizzle of olive oil
- Juice from 1 lime
- Salt and ground black pepper, to taste

For the guacamole:

- 2 avocados, pitted, peeled, and chopped
- Fresh coriander, chopped
- 2 red chilies, chopped
- 1 tomato, cored and chopped
- 1 onion, peeled and chopped
- Juice from 2 limes

Directions:
Season the squid and tentacles with salt, pepper, drizzle some olive oil, and massage well. Place on preheated grill over medium-high heat score side down, and cook for 2 minutes. Flip and cook for 2 minutes, and transfer to a bowl. Add the juice from 1 lime, toss to coat, and keep warm. Put the avocado in a bowl and mash using a fork. Add the coriander, chilies, tomato, onion, and juice from 2 limes, and stir well everything.
Divide the squid on plates, top with guacamole, and serve.

Nutrition: Calories - 500, Fat - 43, Fiber - 6, Carbs - 7, Protein - 20

Shrimp and Cauliflower

Preparation time: 10 minutes
Cooking time: 15 minutes
Servings: 2

Ingredients:

- 1 tablespoon butter
- 1 cauliflower head, separated into florets
- 1 pound shrimp, peeled and deveined
- ¼ cup coconut milk
- 8 ounces mushrooms, chopped
- A pinch of red pepper flakes
- Salt and ground black pepper, to taste
- 2 garlic cloves, peeled and minced
- 4 bacon slices
- ½ cup beef stock
- 1 tablespoon fresh parsley, diced
- 1 tablespoon fresh chives, chopped

Directions:
Heat up a pan over medium-high heat, add the bacon, cook until crispy, transfer to paper towels, and leave aside. Heat up another pan with 1 tablespoon bacon fat over medium-high heat, add the shrimp, cook for 2 minutes on each side, and transfer to a bowl. Heat up the pan again over medium heat, add the mushrooms, stir, and cook for 3-4 minutes. Add the garlic and pepper flakes, stir, and cook for 1 minute. Add the beef stock, salt, pepper, and return shrimp to pan as well. Stir, cook until everything thickens a bit, take off the heat, and keep warm. Meanwhile, put cauliflower in a food processor, and mince it. Place this into a heated pan over medium-high heat, stir, and cook for 5 minutes. Add the butter and butter, stir, and blend using an immersion blender. Add the salt and pepper to taste, stir, and divide into bowls. Top with shrimp mixture, and serve with parsley and chives.

Nutrition: Calories - 245, Fat - 7, Fiber - 4, Carbs - 6, Protein - 20

Salmon Stuffed with Shrimp

Preparation time: 10 minutes
Cooking time: 25 minutes
Servings: 2

Ingredients:
- 2 salmon fillets
- A drizzle of olive oil
- 5 ounces tiger shrimp, peeled, deveined, and chopped
- 6 mushrooms, chopped
- 3 green onions, chopped
- 2 cups spinach
- ¼ cup macadamia nuts, toasted and chopped
- Salt and ground black pepper, to taste
- A pinch of nutmeg
- ¼ cup mayonnaise

Directions:
Heat up a pan with the oil over medium-high heat, add the mushrooms, onions, salt, and pepper, stir, and cook for 4 minutes. Add the macadamia nuts, stir, and cook for 2 minutes. Add the spinach, stir, and cook for 1 minute. Add the shrimp, stir, and cook for 1 minutes. Take off heat, set aside for a few minutes, add the mayonnaise, and nutmeg, and stir well. Make an incision lengthwise in each salmon fillet, sprinkle salt, and pepper, divide the spinach and shrimp mixture into incisions, and place on a working surface. Heat up a pan with a drizzle of oil over medium-high heat, add the stuffed salmon, skin side down, cook for 1 minutes, reduce temperature, cover pan, and cook for 8 minutes. Broil for 3 minutes, divide on plates, and serve.

Nutrition: Calories - 430, Fat - 30, Fiber - 3, Carbs - 7, Protein - 50

Mustard-glazed Salmon

Preparation time: 10 minutes
Cooking time: 20 minutes
Servings: 1

Ingredients:
- 1 salmon fillet
- Salt and ground black pepper, to taste
- 2 tablespoons mustard
- 1 tablespoon coconut oil
- 1 tablespoon maple extract

Directions:
In a bowl, mix the maple extract with the mustard, and whisk. Season the salmon with salt and pepper, and brush the salmon with half of the mustard mixture. Heat up a pan with the oil over medium-high heat, place the salmon flesh side down, and cook for 5 minutes. Brush the salmon with the rest of the mustard mixture, transfer to a baking dish, place in an oven at 425°F, bake for 15 minutes, and serve.

Nutrition: Calories - 240, Fat - 7, Fiber - 1, Carbs - 5, Protein - 23

Salmon with Arugula and Cabbage

Preparation time: 10 minutes
Cooking time: 15 minutes
Servings: 4

Ingredients:
- 3 cups ice water
- 2 teaspoons sriracha sauce
- 4 teaspoons stevia
- 3 scallions, chopped
- Salt and ground black pepper, to taste
- 2 teaspoons flaxseed oil
- 4 teaspoons apple cider vinegar
- 3 teaspoons avocado oil
- 4 medium salmon fillets
- 4 cups baby arugula
- 2 cups cabbage, shredded
- 1½ teaspoon Jamaican jerk seasoning
- ¼ cup sunflower seeds, toasted
- 2 cups watermelon radish, julienned

Directions:
Put ice water in a bowl, add the scallions, and set aside. In another bowl, mix the sriracha sauce with stevia, and stir well. Transfer 2 teaspoons of this mixture to a bowl, and mix with half of the avocado oil, flaxseed oil, vinegar, salt, and pepper, and whisk. Sprinkle the jerk seasoning over the salmon, rub with sriracha, and stevia mixture, and season with salt, and pepper. Heat up a pan with the rest of the avocado oil over medium-high heat, add the salmon, flesh side down, cook for 4 minutes, flip, and cook for 4 minutes, and divide on plates. In a bowl, mix the radishes with cabbage, and arugula. Add the salt, pepper, sriracha, and vinegar mixture, and toss well. Add this to salmon fillets, drizzle the remaining sriracha, and stevia sauce all over, and top with sunflower seeds and drained scallions.

Nutrition: Calories - 160, Fat - 6, Fiber - 1, Carbs - 1, Protein - 12

Scallops with Fennel Sauce

Preparation time: 10 minutes
Cooking time: 10 minutes
Servings: 2

Ingredients:
- 6 scallops
- 1 fennel bulb, trimmed, leaves chopped, and cut into wedges
- Juice of ½ lime
- 1 lime, cut into wedges
- Zest from 1 lime
- 1 egg yolk
- 3 tablespoons butter, melted, and heated up
- ½ tablespoons olive oil
- Salt and ground black pepper, to taste

Directions:
Season the scallops with salt, and pepper, put in a bowl, and mix with half of the lime juice, and half of the zest, and toss to coat. In a bowl, mix the egg yolk with some salt and pepper and the rest of the lime juice and lime zest, and whisk. Add the melted butter and fennel wedges and stir. Brush the fennel wedges with oil, place on heated grill over medium-high heat, cook for 2 minutes, flip, and cook for 2 minutes. Add the scallops on the grill, cook for 2 minutes, flip, and cook for 2 minutes. Divide the fennel, and scallops on plates, drizzle fennel, and butter mixture, and serve with lime wedges on the side.

Nutrition: Calories - 400, Fat - 24, Fiber - 4, Carbs - 12, Protein - 25

Salmon with Lemon Relish

Preparation time: 10 minutes
Cooking time: 1 hour
Servings: 2

Ingredients:
- 2 medium salmon fillets
- Salt and ground black pepper, to taste
- A drizzle of olive oil
- 1 shallot, peeled and chopped
- 1 tablespoon lemon juice
- 1 lemon
- ¼ cup olive oil
- 2 tablespoons fresh parsley, diced

Directions:
Brush the salmon fillets with a drizzle of olive oil, sprinkle with salt and pepper, place on a lined baking sheet, place in an oven at 400°F, and bake for 1 hour. Meanwhile, put the shallot in a bowl, add the 1 tablespoon lemon juice, salt, and pepper, stir, and set aside for 10 minutes. Cut the lemon into thin wedges. Add this to shallots with the parsley and ¼ cup olive oil, and stir. Take the salmon out of the oven, break into medium pieces, and serve with the lemon relish on the side.

Nutrition: Calories - 200, Fat - 10, Fiber - 1, Carbs - 5, Protein - 20

Mussel Soup

Preparation time: 10 minutes
Cooking time: 15 minutes
Servings: 6

Ingredients:
- 2 pounds mussels
- 28 ounces canned crushed tomatoes
- 28 ounces canned diced tomatoes
- 2 cup chicken stock
- 1 teaspoon red pepper flakes
- 3 garlic cloves, peeled and minced
- ½ cup fresh parsley, chopped
- 1 onion, peeled and chopped
- Salt and ground black pepper, to taste
- 1 tablespoon olive oil

Directions:
Heat up a Dutch oven with the oil over medium-high heat, add the onion, stir, and cook for 3 minutes. Add the garlic and red pepper flakes, stir, and cook for 1 minute. Add the tomatoes and stir. Add the chicken stock, salt, and pepper, stir, and bring to a boil. Add the rinsed mussels, salt, and pepper, cook until they open, discard any unopened ones, and mix with parsley. Stir, divide into bowls, and serve.

Nutrition: Calories - 250, Fat - 3, Fiber - 3, Carbs - 2, Protein - 8

Swordfish with Mango Salsa

Preparation time: 10 minutes
Cooking time: 6 minutes
Servings: 2

Ingredients:
- 2 medium swordfish steaks
- Salt and ground black pepper, to taste
- 2 teaspoons avocado oil
- 1 tablespoon fresh cilantro, chopped
- 1 mango, chopped
- 1 avocado, pitted, peeled, and chopped
- A pinch of cumin
- A pinch of onion powder
- A pinch of garlic powder
- 1 orange, peeled and sliced
- ½ balsamic vinegar

Directions:
Season the fish steaks with salt, pepper, garlic powder, onion powder, and cumin. Heat up a pan with half of the oil over medium-high heat, add the fish steaks, and cook them for 3 minutes on each side. In a bowl, mix the avocado with mango, cilantro, balsamic vinegar, salt, pepper, and the rest of the oil, and stir well. Divide fish on plates, top with mango salsa, and serve with orange slices on the side.

Nutrition: Calories - 160, Fat - 3, Fiber - 2, Carbs - 4, Protein - 8

Sushi Bowl

Preparation time: 10 minutes
Cooking time: 7 minutes
Servings: 4

Ingredients:
- 1 ahi tuna steak
- 2 tablespoons coconut oil
- 1 cauliflower head, separated into florets
- 2 tablespoons green onions, chopped
- 1 avocado, pitted, peeled, and chopped
- 1 cucumber, grated
- 1 nori sheet, torn
- Bean sprouts

For the salad dressing:
- 1 tablespoon sesame oil
- 2 tablespoons coconut aminos
- 1 tablespoon apple cider vinegar
- A pinch of salt
- 1 teaspoon stevia

Directions:
Put the cauliflower florets in a food processor and blend until you obtain a cauliflower "rice." Put some water in a pot, put a steamer basket inside, add the cauliflower rice, bring to a boil over medium heat, cover, steam for a few minutes, drain, and transfer the "rice" to a bowl. Heat up a pan with the coconut oil over medium-high heat, add the tuna, cook for 1 minute on each side, and transfer to a cutting board. Divide the cauliflower rice into bowls, top with nori pieces, cloves sprouts, cucumber, green onions, and avocado. In a bowl, mix the sesame oil with vinegar, coconut aminos, salt, and stevia, and whisk. Drizzle this over cauliflower rice and mixed vegetables, top with tuna pieces, and serve.

Nutrition: Calories - 300, Fat - 12, Fiber - 6, Carbs - 6, Protein - 15

Grilled Swordfish

Preparation time: 3 hours and 10 minutes
Cooking time: 10 minutes
Servings: 4

Ingredients:
- 1 tablespoon fresh parsley, chopped
- 1 lemon, cut into wedges
- 4 swordfish steaks
- 3 garlic cloves, peeled and minced
- ⅓ cup chicken stock
- 3 tablespoons olive oil
- ¼ cup lemon juice
- Salt and ground black pepper, to taste
- ½ teaspoon dried rosemary
- ½ teaspoon dried sage
- ½ teaspoon dried marjoram

Directions:
In a bowl, mix the chicken stock with garlic, lemon juice, olive oil, salt, pepper, sage, marjoram, and rosemary, and whisk. Add the swordfish steaks, toss to coat, and keep in the refrigerator for 3 hours. Place the marinated fish steaks on preheated grill over medium-high heat, and cook for 5 minutes on each side. Arrange on plates, sprinkle parsley onto the fish, and serve with lemon wedges on the side.

Nutrition: Calories - 136, Fat - 5, Fiber - 0, Carbs - 1, Protein - 20

Ketogenic Poultry Recipes

Chicken Nuggets

Preparation time: 10 minutes
Cooking time: 15 minutes
Servings: 2

Ingredients:
- ½ cup coconut flour
- 1 egg
- 2 tablespoons garlic powder
- 2 chicken breasts, cubed
- Salt and ground black pepper, to taste
- ½ cup butter

Directions:
In a bowl, mix the garlic powder with the coconut flour, salt, and pepper, and stir. In another bowl, whisk the egg well. Dip the chicken breast cubes in egg mixture, then in flour mixture. Heat up a pan with the butter over medium heat, drop the chicken nuggets, and cook them for 5 minutes on each side. Transfer to paper towels, drain the grease, and then serve.

Nutrition: Calories - 60, Fat - 3, Fiber - 0. 2, Carbs - 3, Protein - 4

Chicken Wings with Mint Chutney

Preparation time: 20 minutes
Cooking time: 25 minutes
Servings: 6

Ingredients:
- 18 chicken wings, cut in half
- 1 tablespoon turmeric
- 1 tablespoon cumin
- 1 tablespoon fresh ginger, grated
- 1 tablespoon coriander
- 1 tablespoon paprika
- A pinch of cayenne pepper
- Salt and ground black pepper, to taste
- 2 tablespoons olive oil

For the chutney:
- Juice of ½ lime
- 1 cup fresh mint leaves
- 1 small ginger piece, peeled and chopped
- ¾ cup cilantro
- 1 tablespoon olive oil
- 1 tablespoon water
- Salt and ground black pepper, to taste
- 1 Serrano pepper

Directions:
In a bowl, mix the 1 tablespoon ginger with cumin, coriander, paprika, turmeric, salt, pepper, cayenne, and 2 tablespoons oil, and stir well. Add the chicken wings pieces to this mixture, toss to coat well, and keep in the refrigerator for 20 minutes. Heat up a grill over high heat, add the marinated wings, cook for 25 minutes, turning them from time to time, and transfer to a bowl. In a blender, mix the mint with cilantro, ginger, juice from ½ lime, 1 tablespoon olive oil, salt, pepper, water, and Serrano pepper, and blend well. Serve the chicken wings with this sauce on the side.

Nutrition: Calories - 100, Fat - 5, Fiber - 1, Carbs - 1, Protein - 9

Chicken Meatballs

Preparation time: 10 minutes
Cooking time: 15 minutes
Servings: 3

Ingredients:
- 1 pound ground chicken
- Salt and ground black pepper, to taste
- 2 tablespoons ranch dressing
- ½ cup almond flour
- ¼ cup cheddar cheese, grated
- 1 tablespoon dry ranch seasoning
- ¼ cup hot sauce + more for serving
- 1 egg

Directions:
In a bowl, mix the chicken meat with salt, pepper, ranch dressing, flour, dry ranch seasoning, cheddar cheese, hot sauce, and the egg, and stir well. Shape 9 meatballs, place them on a lined baking sheet, and bake at 500ºF for 15 minutes. Serve the chicken meatballs with hot sauce on the side.

Nutrition: Calories - 156, Fat - 11, Fiber - 1, Carbs - 2, Protein - 12

Grilled Chicken Wings

Preparation time: 2 hours and 10 minutes
Cooking time: 15 minutes
Servings: 5

Ingredients:
- 2 pounds wings
- Juice from 1 lime
- ½ cup fresh cilantro, chopped
- 2 garlic cloves, peeled and minced
- 1 jalapeño pepper, chopped
- 3 tablespoons coconut oil
- Salt and ground black pepper, to taste
- Lime wedges, for serving
- Ranch dip, for serving

Directions:
In a bowl, mix the lime juice with the cilantro, garlic, jalapeño, coconut oil, salt, and pepper, and whisk. Add the chicken wings, toss to coat, and keep in the refrigerator for 2 hours. Place the chicken wings on a preheated grill over medium-high heat, and cook for 7 minutes on each side. Serve the chicken wings with ranch dip and lime wedges.

Nutrition: Calories - 132, Fat - 5, Fiber - 1, Carbs - 4, Protein - 12

Easy Baked Chicken

Preparation time: 10 minutes
Cooking time: 20 minutes
Servings: 4

Ingredients:
- 4 bacon strips
- 4 chicken breasts
- 3 green onions, chopped
- 4 ounces ranch dressing
- 1 ounce coconut aminos
- 2 tablespoons coconut oil
- 4 ounces cheddar cheese, grated

Directions:
Heat up a pan with the oil over high heat, add the chicken breasts, cook for 7 minutes, flip, and cook for 7 more minutes. Heat up another pan over medium-high heat, add the bacon, cook until crispy, transfer to paper towels, drain the grease, and crumble. Transfer the chicken breast to a baking dish, add the coconut aminos, crumbled bacon, cheese, and green onions on top, introduce in an oven, set on broiler, and cook at a high temperature for 5 minutes. Divide on plates and serve.

Nutrition: Calories - 450, Fat - 24, Fiber - 0, Carbs - 3, Protein - 60

Italian Chicken

Preparation time: 10 minutes
Cooking time: 20 minutes
Servings: 4

Ingredients:
- ¼ cup olive oil
- 1 onion, peeled and chopped
- 4 chicken breasts, skinless and boneless
- 4 garlic cloves, peeled and minced
- Salt and ground black pepper, to taste
- ½ cup green olives, pitted and chopped
- 4 anchovy fillets, chopped
- 1 tablespoon capers, chopped
- 1 pound tomatoes, cored and chopped
- ½ teaspoon red chili flakes

Directions:
Season the chicken with salt, and pepper, and rub with half of the oil. Place into a pan which you've heated over high temperature, cook for 2 minutes, flip, and cook for 2 minutes. Place the chicken breasts in the oven at 450ºF and bake for 8 minutes. Take the chicken out of the oven and divide on plates. Heat up the same pan with the rest of the oil over medium heat, add the onion, garlic, olives, anchovies, chili flakes, and capers, stir, and cook for 1 minute. Add the salt, pepper, and tomatoes, stir, and cook for 2 minutes. Drizzle this over chicken breasts and serve.

Nutrition: Calories - 400, Fat - 20, Fiber - 1, Carbs - 2, Protein - 7

Lemon Chicken

Preparation time: 10 minutes
Cooking time: 45 minutes
Servings: 6

Ingredients:
- 1 whole chicken, cut into medium-sized pieces
- Salt and ground black pepper, to taste
- Juice from 2 lemons
- Zest from 2 lemons
- Lemon rinds from 2 lemons

Directions:
Put the chicken pieces in a baking dish, season with some salt and pepper, and drizzle lemon juice. Toss to coat well, add the lemon zest, and lemon rinds, place in an oven at 375ºF, and bake for 45 minutes. Discard the lemon rinds, divide the chicken onto plates, drizzle sauce from the baking dish over it, and serve.

Nutrition: Calories - 334, Fat - 24, Fiber - 2, Carbs - 4. 5, Protein - 27

Fried Chicken with Paprika Sauce

Preparation time: 10 minutes
Cooking time: 20 minutes
Servings: 5

Ingredients:
- 1 tablespoon coconut oil
- 3½ pounds chicken breasts
- 1 cup chicken stock
- 1¼ cups onion, peeled and chopped
- 1 tablespoon lime juice
- ¼ cup coconut milk
- 2 teaspoons paprika
- 1 teaspoon red pepper flakes
- 2 tablespoons green onions, chopped
- Salt and ground black pepper, to taste

Directions:
Heat up a pan with the oil over medium-high heat, add the chicken, cook for 2 minutes on each side, transfer to a plate, and set aside. Reduce heat to medium, add the onions to the pan, and cook for 4 minutes. Add the stock, coconut milk, pepper flakes, paprika, lime juice, salt, and pepper, and stir well. Return the chicken to the pan, add more salt, and pepper, cover the pan, and cook for 15 minutes. Divide on plates and serve.

Nutrition: Calories - 140, Fat - 4, Fiber - 3, Carbs - 3, Protein - 6

Chicken Fajitas

Preparation time: 10 minutes
Cooking time: 15 minutes
Servings: 4

Ingredients:
- 2 pounds chicken breasts, skinless, boneless, and cut into strips
- 1 teaspoon garlic powder
- 1 teaspoon chili powder
- 2 teaspoons cumin
- 2 tablespoons lime juice
- Salt and ground black pepper, to taste
- 1 teaspoon sweet paprika
- 2 tablespoons coconut oil
- 1 teaspoon coriander
- 1 green bell pepper, seeded and sliced
- 1 red bell pepper, seeded and sliced
- 1 onion, peeled and sliced
- 1 tablespoon fresh cilantro, chopped
- 1 avocado, pitted, peeled, and sliced
- 2 limes, cut into wedges

Directions:
In a bowl, mix the lime juice with the chili powder, cumin, salt, pepper, garlic powder, paprika, and coriander, and stir. Add the chicken pieces and toss to coat well. Heat up a pan with half of the oil over medium-high heat, add the chicken, cook for 3 minutes on each side, and transfer to a bowl. Heat up the pan with the rest of the oil over medium heat, add the onion and bell peppers, stir, and cook for 6 minutes. Return the chicken to pan, add more salt, and pepper, stir, and divide on plates. Top with avocado, lime wedges, and cilantro, and serve.

Nutrition: Calories - 240, Fat - 10, Fiber - 2, Carbs - 5, Protein - 20

Skillet Chicken and Mushrooms

Preparation time: 10 minutes
Cooking time: 30 minutes
Servings: 4

Ingredients:
- 4 chicken thighs
- 2 cups mushrooms, sliced
- ¼ cup butter
- Salt and ground black pepper, to taste
- ½ teaspoon onion powder
- ½ teaspoon garlic powder
- ½ cup water
- 1 teaspoon Dijon mustard
- 1 tablespoon fresh tarragon, chopped

Directions:
Heat up a pan with half of the butter over medium-high heat, add the chicken thighs, season them with salt, pepper, garlic powder, and onion powder, cook the for 3 minutes on each side, and transfer to a bowl. Heat up the same pan with the rest of the butter over medium-high heat, add the mushrooms, stir, and cook for 5 minutes. Add the mustard and water, and stir well. Return the chicken pieces to the pan, stir, cover, and cook for 15 minutes. Add the tarragon, stir, cook for 5 minutes, divide on plates, and serve.

Nutrition: Calories - 453, Fat - 32, Fiber - 6, Carbs - 1, Protein - 36

Chicken with Olive Tapenade

Preparation time: 10 minutes
Cooking time: 10 minutes
Servings: 2

Ingredients:
- 1 chicken breast, cut into 4 pieces
- 2 tablespoons coconut oil
- 3 garlic cloves, peeled, and crushed
- ½ cup olives tapenade

For the tapenade:
- 1 cup black olives, pitted
- Salt and ground black pepper, to taste
- 2 tablespoons olive oil
- ¼ cup fresh parsley, chopped
- 1 tablespoons lemon juice

Directions:
In a food processor, mix the olives with salt, pepper, 2 tablespoons olive oil, lemon juice, and parsley, blend well, and transfer to a bowl. Heat up a pan with the coconut oil over medium heat, add the garlic, stir, and cook for 2 minutes. Add the chicken pieces and cook for 4 minutes on each side. Divide chicken on plates and top with the olives tapenade.

Nutrition: Calories - 130, Fat - 12, Fiber - 0, Carbs - 3, Protein - 20

Pan-seared Duck Breast

Preparation time: 10 minutes
Cooking time: 20 minutes
Servings: 1

Ingredients:
- 1 medium duck breast, skin scored
- 1 tablespoon swerve
- 1 tablespoon heavy cream
- 2 tablespoons butter
- ½ teaspoon orange extract
- Salt and ground black pepper, to taste
- 1 cup baby spinach
- ¼ teaspoon fresh sage

Directions:
Heat up a pan with the butter over medium heat. Once it melts, add the swerve and stir until butter browns. Add the orange extract and sage, stir, and cook for 2 minutes. Add the heavy cream and stir again. Heat up another pan over medium-high heat, add the duck breast, skin side down, cook for 4 minutes, flip, and cook for another 3 minutes. Pour the orange sauce over duck breast, stir, and cook for a few minutes. Add the spinach to the pan with the sauce, stir, and cook for 1 minute. Take the duck off heat, slice the duck breast, and arrange on a plate. Drizzle the orange sauce on top and serve with the spinach on the side.

Nutrition: Calories - 567, Fat - 56, Fiber - 0, Carbs - 0, Protein - 35

Duck Breast with Vegetables

Preparation time: 10 minutes
Cooking time: 10 minutes
Servings: 2

Ingredients:
- 2 duck breasts, skin on and sliced thin
- 2 zucchini, sliced
- 1 tablespoon coconut oil
- 1 green onion bunch, chopped
- 1 daikon, chopped
- 2 green bell peppers, seeded and chopped
- Salt and ground black pepper, to taste

Directions:
Heat up a pan with the oil over medium-high heat, add the green onions, stir, and cook for 2 minutes. Add the zucchini, daikon, bell peppers, salt, and pepper, stir, and cook for 10 minutes. Heat up another pan over medium-high heat, add the duck slices, cook for 3 minutes on each side, and transfer to the pan with the vegetables. Cook for 3 minutes, divide on plates, and serve.

Nutrition: Calories - 450, Fat - 23, Fiber - 3, Carbs - 8, Protein - 50

Duck Breast Salad

Preparation time: 10 minutes
Cooking time: 15 minutes
Servings: 4

Ingredients:
- 1 tablespoon swerve
- 1 shallot, peeled and chopped
- ¼ cup red vinegar
- ¼ cup olive oil
- ¼ cup water
- ¾ cup raspberries
- 1 tablespoon Dijon mustard
- Salt and ground black pepper, to taste

For the salad:
- 10 ounces baby spinach
- 2 medium duck breasts, boneless
- 4 ounces goat cheese, crumbled
- Salt and ground black pepper, to taste
- ½ pint raspberries
- ½ cup pecans halves

Directions:
In a blender, mix the swerve with shallot, vinegar, water, oil, ¾ cup raspberries, mustard, salt, and pepper, and blend well. Strain this into a bowl, and leave aside. Score the duck breast, season with salt, and pepper, and place skin side down into a pan heated up over medium-high heat. Cook for 8 minutes, flip, and cook for 5 minutes. Divide the spinach on plates, sprinkle with the goat cheese, pecan halves, and ½ pint raspberries. Slice the duck breasts and add on top of raspberries. Drizzle the raspberries vinaigrette on top and serve.

Nutrition: Calories - 455, Fat - 40, Fiber - 4, Carbs - 6, Protein - 18

Turkey Pie

Preparation time: 10 minutes
Cooking time: 40 minutes
Servings: 6

Ingredients:
- 2 cups turkey stock
- 1 cup turkey meat, cooked and shredded
- Salt and ground black pepper, to taste
- 1 teaspoon fresh thyme, chopped
- ½ cup kale, chopped
- ½ cup butternut squash, peeled and chopped
- ½ cup cheddar cheese, shredded
- ¼ teaspoon paprika
- ¼ teaspoon garlic powder
- ¼ teaspoon xanthan gum
- Vegetable oil cooking spray

For the crust:
- ¼ cup butter
- ¼ teaspoon xanthan gum
- 2 cups almond flour
- A pinch of salt
- 1 egg
- ¼ cup cheddar cheese

Directions:
Heat up a pot with the stock over medium heat. Add the squash and turkey meat, stir, and cook for 10 minutes. Add the garlic powder, kale, thyme, paprika, salt, pepper, and ½ cup cheddar cheese, and stir well. In a bowl, mix the ¼ teaspoon xanthan gum with ½ cup stock from the pot, stir well, and add everything to the pot. Take off the heat and set aside. In a bowl, mix the flour with ¼ teaspoon xanthan gum and a pinch of salt and stir. Add the butter, egg, ¼ cup cheddar cheese, and stir until a pie crust dough forms. Shape into a ball and place it in the refrigerator. Spray a baking dish with cooking spray and spread pie filling on the bottom. Transfer dough to a working surface, roll into a circle, and top filling with this. Press well, and seal edges, place in an oven at 350ºF, and bake for 35 minutes. Let the pie to cool, and serve.

Nutrition: Calories - 320, Fat - 23, Fiber - 8, Carbs - 6, Protein - 16

Turkey Soup

Preparation time: 10 minutes
Cooking time: 30 minutes
Servings: 4

Ingredients:
- 3 celery stalks, chopped
- 1 onion, peeled and chopped
- 1 tablespoon butter
- 6 cups turkey stock
- Salt and ground black pepper, to taste
- ¼ cup fresh parsley, chopped
- 3 cups baked spaghetti squash, chopped
- 3 cups turkey, cooked, and shredded

Directions:
Heat up a pot with the butter over medium-high heat, add the celery and onion, stir, and cook for 5 minutes. Add the parsley, stock, turkey meat, salt, and pepper, stir, and cook for 20 minutes. Add the spaghetti squash, stir, and cook turkey soup for 10 minutes. Divide into bowls and serve.

Nutrition: Calories - 150, Fat - 4, Fiber - 1, Carbs - 3, Protein - 10

Baked Turkey Delight

Preparation time: 10 minutes
Cooking time: 45 minutes
Servings: 8

Ingredients:
- 4 cups zucchini, cut with a spiralizer
- 1 egg, whisked
- 3 cups cabbage, shredded
- 3 cups turkey meat, cooked and shredded
- ½ cup turkey stock
- ½ cup cream cheese
- 1 teaspoon poultry seasoning
- 2 cup cheddar cheese, grated
- ½ cup Parmesan cheese, grated
- Salt and ground black pepper, to taste
- ¼ teaspoon garlic powder

Directions:
Heat up a pan with the stock over medium-low heat. Add the egg, cream, Parmesan cheese, cheddar cheese, salt, pepper, poultry seasoning, and garlic powder, stir, and bring to a gentle simmer. Add the turkey meat, and cabbage, stir, and take off the heat. Place the zucchini noodles in a baking dish, add the some salt and pepper, add the turkey mixture, and spread. Cover with aluminum foil, place in an oven at 400°F, and bake for 35 minutes. Set aside to cool before serving.

Nutrition: Calories - 240, Fat - 15, Fiber - 1, Carbs - 3, Protein - 25

Turkey Chili

Preparation time: 10 minutes
Cooking time: 20 minutes
Servings: 8

Ingredients:
- 4 cups turkey meat, cooked and shredded
- 2 cups squash, chopped
- 6 cups chicken stock
- Salt and ground black pepper, to taste
- 1 tablespoon canned chipotle peppers, chopped
- ½ teaspoon garlic powder
- ½ cup salsa verde
- 1 teaspoon coriander
- 2 teaspoons cumin
- ¼ cup sour cream
- 1 tablespoon fresh cilantro, chopped

Directions:
Heat up a pan with the stock over medium heat. Add the squash, stir, and cook for 10 minutes. Add the turkey, chipotles, garlic powder, salsa verde, cumin, coriander, salt, and pepper, stir, and cook for 10 minutes. Add the sour cream, stir, take off the heat, and divide into bowls. Top with some chopped cilantro and serve.

Nutrition: Calories - 154, Fat - 5, Fiber - 3, Carbs - 2, Protein - 27

Turkey and Tomato Curry

Preparation time: 10 minutes
Cooking time: 20 minutes
Servings: 4

Ingredients:
- 18 ounces turkey meat, minced
- 3 ounces spinach
- 20 ounces canned diced tomatoes
- 2 tablespoons coconut oil
- 2 tablespoons coconut cream
- 2 garlic cloves, peeled and minced
- 2 onions, peeled, and sliced
- 1 tablespoon coriander
- 2 tablespoons fresh ginger, grated
- 1 tablespoons turmeric
- 1 tablespoon cumin
- Salt and ground black pepper, to taste
- 2 tablespoons chili powder

Directions:
Heat up a pan with the coconut oil over medium heat, add the onion, stir, and cook for 5 minutes. Add the ginger and garlic, stir, and cook for 1 minute. Add the tomatoes, salt, pepper, coriander, cumin, turmeric, and chili powder, and stir. Add the coconut cream, stir, and cook for 10 minutes. Blend using an immersion blender and mix with spinach and turkey meat. Bring to a simmer, cook for 15 minutes, and serve.

Nutrition: Calories - 240, Fat - 4, Fiber - 3, Carbs - 2, Protein - 12

Turkey and Cranberry Salad

Preparation time: 10 minutes
Cooking time: 0 minutes
Servings: 4

Ingredients:
- 4 cups romaine lettuce leaves, torn
- 2 cups turkey breast, cooked and cubed
- 1 orange, peeled, and cut into small segments
- 1 red apple, cored and chopped
- 3 tablespoons walnuts, chopped
- 3 kiwis, peeled and sliced
- ¼ cup cranberries
- 1 cup cranberry sauce
- 1 cup orange juice

Directions:
In a salad bowl, mix the lettuce with turkey, orange segments, apple pieces, cranberries, and walnuts, and toss to coat. In another bowl, mix the cranberry sauce and orange juice, and stir. Drizzle this over turkey salad, toss to coat, and serve with the kiwis on top.

Nutrition: Calories - 120, Fat - 2, Fiber - 1, Carbs - 3, Protein - 7

Stuffed Chicken Breast

Preparation time: 10 minutes
Cooking time: 15 minutes
Servings: 3

Ingredients:
- 8 ounces spinach, cooked, and chopped
- 3 chicken breasts
- Salt and ground black pepper, to taste
- 4 ounces cream cheese, softened
- 3 ounces feta cheese, crumbled
- 1 garlic clove, peeled and minced
- 1 tablespoon coconut oil

Directions:
In a bowl, mix the feta cheese with cream cheese, spinach, salt, pepper, and the garlic, and stir well. Place the chicken breasts on a working surface, cut a pocket in each, stuff them with the spinach mixture, and season them with some salt and pepper. Heat up a pan with the oil over medium-high heat, add the stuffed chicken, cook for 5 minutes on each side, and then place in the oven at 450°F. Bake for 10 minutes, divide on plates, and serve.

Nutrition: Calories - 290, Fat - 12, Fiber - 2, Carbs - 4, Protein - 24

Chicken with Mustard Sauce

Preparation time: 10 minutes
Cooking time: 30 minutes
Servings: 3

Ingredients:
- 8 bacon strips, chopped
- ⅓ cup Dijon mustard
- Salt and ground black pepper, to taste
- 1 cup onion, chopped
- 1 tablespoon olive oil
- 1½ cups chicken stock
- 3 chicken breasts, skinless and boneless
- ¼ teaspoon sweet paprika

Directions:
In a bowl, mix the paprika with the mustard, salt, and pepper, and stir well. Spread this on chicken breasts and massage. Heat up a pan over medium-high heat, add the bacon, stir, cook until it browns, and transfer to a plate. Heat up the same pan with the oil over medium-high heat, add the chicken breasts, cook for 2 minutes on each side, and transfer to a plate. Heat up the pan once again over medium-high heat, add the stock, stir, and bring to a simmer. Add the bacon and onions, salt, and pepper, and stir. Return the chicken to pan as well, stir gently, and simmer over medium heat for 20 minutes, turning the meat halfway through. Divide the chicken on plates, drizzle the sauce over it, and serve.

Nutrition: Calories - 223, Fat - 8, Fiber - 1, Carbs - 3, Protein - 26

Salsa Chicken

Preparation time: 10 minutes
Cooking time: 1 hour and 15 minutes
Servings: 6

Ingredients:
- 6 chicken breasts, skinless and boneless
- 2 cups jarred salsa
- Salt and ground black pepper, to taste
- 1 cup cheddar cheese, shredded
- Vegetable cooking spray

Directions:
Spray a baking dish with cooking oil, place chicken breasts on it, season with salt, and pepper, and pour salsa all over. Place in an oven at 425°F, and bake for 1 hour. Spread cheese, and bake for 15 minutes. Divide on plates and serve.

Nutrition: Calories - 120, Fat - 2, Fiber - 2, Carbs - 6, Protein - 10

Italian Chicken

Preparation time: 10 minutes
Cooking time: 1 hour
Servings: 6

Ingredients:
- 8 ounces mushrooms, chopped
- 1 pound Italian sausage, chopped
- 2 tablespoons avocado oil
- 6 cherry peppers, chopped
- 1 red bell pepper, seeded and chopped
- 1 onion, peeled and sliced
- 2 tablespoons garlic, minced
- 2 cups cherry tomatoes, halved
- 4 chicken thighs
- Salt and ground black pepper, to taste
- ½ cup chicken stock
- 1 tablespoon balsamic vinegar
- 2 teaspoons dried oregano
- Fresh parsley, chopped, for serving

Directions:
Heat up a pan with half of the oil over medium heat, add the sausages, stir, brown for a few minutes, and transfer to a plate. Heat up the pan again with the rest of the oil over medium heat, add the chicken thighs, season with salt, and pepper, cook for 3 minutes on each side, and transfer to a plate. Heat up the pan again over medium heat, add the cherry peppers, mushrooms, onion, and bell pepper, stir, and cook for 4 minutes. Add the garlic, stir, and cook for 2 minutes. Add the stock, vinegar, salt, pepper, oregano, and cherry tomatoes, and stir. Add the chicken and sausages, stir gently, transfer everything to the oven at 400 degrees, and bake for 30 minutes. Sprinkle the parsley, divide on plates, and serve.

Nutrition: Calories - 340, Fat - 33, Fiber - 3, Carbs - 4, Protein - 20

Chicken Casserole

Preparation time: 10 minutes
Cooking time: 40 minutes
Servings: 8

Ingredients:
- 1½ pounds chicken breast, skinless, boneless, and cubed
- Salt and ground black pepper, to taste
- 1 egg
- 1 cup almond flour
- ¼ cup Parmesan cheese, grated
- ½ teaspoon garlic powder
- 1½ teaspoons dried parsley
- ½ teaspoon dried basil
- 4 tablespoons avocado oil
- 4 cups spaghetti squash, already cooked
- 6 ounces mozzarella cheese, shredded
- 1½ cups keto marinara sauce
- Fresh basil, chopped, for serving

Directions:
In a bowl, mix the almond flour with Parmesan, salt, pepper, garlic powder, and 1 teaspoon parsley, and stir. In another bowl, whisk the egg with a pinch of salt and pepper. Dip the chicken in the egg, and then in almond flour mixture. Heat up a pan with 3 tablespoons oil over medium-high heat, add the chicken, cook until they are golden brown on both sides, and transfer to paper towels. In a bowl, mix the spaghetti squash with salt, pepper, dried basil, 1 tablespoon oil, and the rest of the parsley, and stir. Spread this into a heatproof dish, add the chicken pieces, and then the marinara sauce. Top with the shredded mozzarella cheese, place in an oven at 375°F, and bake for 30 minutes. Sprinkle with fresh basil at the end, set the casserole aside to cool, divide on plates, and serve.

Nutrition: Calories - 300, Fat - 6, Fiber - 3, Carbs - 5, Protein - 28

Chicken-stuffed Peppers

Preparation time: 10 minutes
Cooking time: 40 minutes
Servings: 3

Ingredients:
- 2 cups cauliflower florets
- Salt and ground black pepper, to taste
- 1 onion, peeled and chopped
- 2 chicken breasts, skinless, boneless, cooked, and shredded
- 2 tablespoons fajita seasoning
- 1 tablespoon butter
- 6 bell peppers, tops cut off and seeds removed
- ⅔ cup water

Directions:
Put the cauliflower florets in a food processor, add a pinch of salt and pepper, pulse well, and transfer to a bowl. Heat up a pan with the butter over medium heat, add the onions, stir, and cook for 2 minutes. Add the cauliflower, stir, and cook for 3 minutes. Add the seasoning, salt, pepper, water, and chicken, stir, and cook for 2 minutes. Place the bell peppers on a lined baking sheet, stuff each with chicken mixture, place in an oven at 350°F, and bake for 30 minutes. Divide them on plates and serve.

Nutrition: Calories - 200, Fat - 6, Fiber - 3, Carbs - 6, Protein - 14

Creamy Chicken

Preparation time: 10 minutes
Cooking time: 1 hour
Servings: 4

Ingredients:
- 4 chicken breasts, skinless and boneless
- ½ cup mayonnaise
- ½ cup sour cream
- Salt and ground black pepper, to taste
- ¾ cup Parmesan cheese, grated
- Vegetable oil cooking spray
- 8 mozzarella cheese slices
- 1 teaspoon garlic powder

Directions:
Spray a baking dish, place the chicken breasts in it, and top each piece with 2 mozzarella cheese slices. In a bowl, mix the Parmesan cheese with salt, pepper, mayonnaise, garlic powder, and sour cream, and stir well. Spread this over the chicken, place the dish in the oven at 375°F, and bake for 1 hour. Divide on plates and serve.

Nutrition: Calories - 240, Fat - 4, Fiber - 3, Carbs - 6, Protein - 20

Chicken and Broccoli Casserole

Preparation time: 10 minutes
Cooking time: 45 minutes
Servings: 4

Ingredients:
- 3 cups cheddar cheese, grated
- 10 ounces broccoli florets
- 3 chicken breasts, skinless, boneless, cooked, and cubed
- 1 cup mayonnaise
- 1 tablespoon coconut oil, melted
- ⅓ cup chicken stock
- Salt and ground black pepper, to taste
- Juice of 1 lemon

Directions:
Grease a baking dish with oil, and arrange chicken pieces on the bottom. Spread broccoli florets, and then half of the cheese. In a bowl, mix the mayo with stock, salt, pepper, and lemon juice. Pour this over the chicken, sprinkle the rest of the cheese, cover dish with aluminum foil, and bake in the oven at 350°F for 30 minutes. Remove the aluminum foil, and bake for 20 minutes. Serve hot.

Nutrition: Calories - 250, Fat - 5, Fiber - 4, Carbs - 6, Protein - 25

Creamy Chicken Soup

Preparation time: 10 minutes
Cooking time: 20 minutes
Servings: 4

Ingredients:
- 3 tablespoons butter
- 4 ounces cream cheese
- 2 cups chicken meat, cooked and shredded
- 4 cups chicken stock
- Salt and ground black pepper, to taste
- ½ cup sour cream
- ¼ cup celery, chopped

Directions:
In a blender, mix the stock with the red sauce, cream cheese, butter, salt, pepper, and sour cream, and pulse well. Transfer this to a pot, heat up over medium heat, and add the celery and chicken. Stir, simmer for a few minutes, divide into bowls, and serve.

Nutrition: Calories - 400, Fat - 23, Fiber - 5, Carbs - 5, Protein - 30

Chicken Crepes

Preparation time: 10 minutes
Cooking time: 30 minutes
Servings: 8

Ingredients:
- 6 eggs
- 6 ounces cream cheese
- 1 teaspoon erythritol
- 1½ tablespoons coconut flour
- ⅓ cup Parmesan cheese, grated
- A pinch of xanthan gum
- Vegetable oil cooking spray

For the filling:
- 8 ounces spinach
- 8 ounces mushrooms, sliced
- 8 ounces rotisserie chicken, shredded
- 8 ounces cheese blend
- 2 ounces cream cheese
- 1 garlic clove, peeled and minced
- 1 onion, peeled and chopped

Liquids:
- 2 tablespoons red wine vinegar
- 2 tablespoons butter
- ½ cup heavy cream
- 1 teaspoon Worcestershire sauce
- ¼ cup chicken stock
- A pinch of nutmeg
- Fresh parsley, chopped
- Salt and ground black pepper, to taste

Directions:
In a bowl, mix the 6 ounces cream cheese with eggs, Parmesan cheese, erythritol, xanthan, and coconut flour, and stir well until you obtain a crepe batter. Heat up a pan over medium heat, spray some cooking oil, pour some of the batters, spread well into the pan, cook for 2 minutes, flip, and cook for 30 seconds more. Repeat with the rest of the batter, and place all crepes on a plate. Heat up a pan with 2 tablespoon butter over medium-high heat, add the onion, stir, and cook for 2 minutes. Add the garlic, stir, and cook for 1 minute. Add the mushrooms, stir, and cook for 2 minutes. Add the chicken, spinach, salt, pepper, stock, vinegar, nutmeg, Worcestershire sauce, heavy cream, cream cheese, and 6 ounces of the cheese blend, stir, and cook for 7 minutes. Fill each crepe with this mixture, roll them, and arrange them all in a baking dish. Top with the remaining cheese blend, place under a preheated broiler for a couple of minutes. Divide the crepes on plates, top with chopped parsley, and serve.

Nutrition: Calories - 360, Fat - 32, Fiber - 2, Carbs - 7, Protein - 20

Four-cheese Chicken

Preparation time: 10 minutes
Cooking time: 50 minutes
Servings: 4

Ingredients:
- 3 pounds chicken breasts
- 2 ounces muenster cheese, cubed
- 2 ounces cream cheese
- 4 ounces cheddar cheese, cubed
- 2 ounces provolone cheese, cubed
- 1 zucchini, shredded
- Salt and ground black pepper, to taste
- 1 teaspoon garlic, minced
- ½ cup bacon, cooked and crumbled

Directions:
Season the zucchini with salt and pepper, set aside for a few minutes, squeeze well, and transfer to a bowl. Add the bacon, garlic, more salt, and pepper, cream cheese, cheddar cheese, Muenster cheese, and provolone cheese, and stir. Cut slits into chicken breasts, season with salt, and pepper, and stuff with the zucchini and cheese mixture. Place on a lined baking sheet, place in an oven at 400°F, and bake for 45 minutes. Divide on plates and serve.

Nutrition: Calories - 455, Fat - 20, Fiber - 0, Carbs - 2, Protein - 57

Crusted Chicken

Preparation time: 10 minutes
Cooking time: 35 minutes
Servings: 4

Ingredients:
- 4 bacon slices, cooked and crumbled
- 4 chicken breasts, skinless and boneless
- 1 tablespoon water
- ½ cup avocado oil
- 1 egg, whisked
- Salt and ground black pepper, to taste
- 1 cup Asiago cheese, shredded
- ¼ teaspoon garlic powder
- 1 cup Parmesan cheese, grated

Directions:
In a bowl, mix the Parmesan cheese with garlic, salt, and pepper, and stir. Put the whisked egg in another bowl and mix with the water. Season the chicken with salt, and pepper, and dip each piece into egg, and then into cheese mixture. Heat up a pan with the oil over medium-high heat, add the chicken breasts, cook until they are golden on both sides, and transfer to a baking pan. Place in an oven at 350°F, and bake for 20 minutes. Top the chicken with the bacon and Asiago cheese, place in an oven, turn on broiler, and broil for a couple of minutes. Serve hot.

Nutrition: Calories - 400, Fat - 22, Fiber - 1, Carbs - 1, Protein - 47

Cheesy Chicken

Preparation time: 10 minutes
Cooking time: 30 minutes
Servings: 4

Ingredients:
- 1 zucchini, chopped
- Salt and ground black pepper, to taste
- 1 teaspoon garlic powder
- 1 tablespoon avocado oil
- 2 chicken breasts, skinless, boneless, and sliced
- 1 tomato, cored and chopped
- ½ teaspoon dried oregano
- ½ teaspoon dried basil
- ½ cup mozzarella cheese, shredded

Directions:
Season the chicken with salt, pepper, and garlic powder. Heat up a pan with the oil over medium heat, add the chicken slices, brown on all sides, and transfer them to a baking dish. Heat up the pan again over medium heat, add the zucchini, oregano, tomato, basil, salt, and pepper, stir, cook for 2 minutes, and pour over chicken. Place in an oven at 325°F, and bake for 20 minutes. Spread the mozzarella cheese over the chicken, place in an oven again, and bake for 5 minutes. Divide on plates and serve.

Nutrition: Calories - 235, Fat - 4, Fiber - 1, Carbs - 2, Protein - 35

Orange Chicken

Preparation time: 10 minutes
Cooking time: 15 minutes
Servings: 4

Ingredients:
- 2 pounds chicken thighs, skinless, boneless, and cut into pieces
- Salt and ground black pepper, to taste
- 3 tablespoons coconut oil
- ¼ cup coconut flour

For the sauce:
- 2 tablespoons fish sauce
- 1½ teaspoons orange extract
- 1 tablespoon fresh ginger, grated
- ¼ cup orange juice
- 2 teaspoons stevia
- 1 tablespoon orange zest
- ¼ teaspoon sesame seeds
- 2 tablespoons scallions, chopped
- ½ teaspoon coriander
- 1 cup water
- ¼ teaspoon red pepper flakes
- 2 tablespoons gluten-free soy sauce

Directions:
In a bowl, mix the coconut flour, salt, and pepper, and stir. Add the chicken pieces and toss to coat well. Heat up a pan with the oil over medium heat, add the chicken, cook until golden brown on both sides, and transfer to a bowl. In a blender, mix the orange juice with the ginger, fish sauce, soy sauce, stevia, orange extract, water, and coriander, and blend well. Pour this into a pan and heat up over medium heat. Add the chicken, stir, and cook for 2 minutes. Add the sesame seeds, orange zest, scallions, and pepper flakes, stir cook for 2 minutes, and take off the heat. Divide on plates and serve.

Nutrition: Calories - 423, Fat - 20, Fiber - 5, Carbs - 6, Protein - 45

Chicken Pie

Preparation time: 10 minutes
Cooking time: 45 minutes
Servings: 4

Ingredients:
- ½ cup onion, peeled and chopped
- 3 tablespoons butter
- ½ cup carrots, peeled and chopped
- 3 garlic cloves, peeled and minced
- Salt and ground black pepper, to taste
- ¾ cup heavy cream
- ½ cup chicken stock
- 12 ounces chicken, cubed
- 2 tablespoons Dijon mustard
- ¾ cup cheddar cheese, shredded

For the dough:
- ¾ cup almond flour
- 3 tablespoons cream cheese
- 1½ cup mozzarella cheese, shredded
- 1 egg
- 1 teaspoon onion powder
- 1 teaspoon garlic powder
- 1 teaspoon Italian seasoning
- Salt and ground black pepper, to taste

Directions:
Heat up a pan with the butter over medium heat, add the onion, carrots, garlic, salt, and pepper, stir, and cook for 5 minutes. Add the chicken, stir, and cook for 3 minutes. Add the heavy cream, stock, salt, pepper, and mustard, stir, and cook for 7 minutes. Add the cheddar cheese, stir well, take off the heat, and keep warm. In a bowl, mix the mozzarella cheese with the cream cheese, stir, and heat up in a microwave for 1 minute. Add the garlic powder, Italian seasoning, salt, pepper, onion powder, flour, and egg, and stir well. Knead the dough well, divide into 4 pieces, and flatten each into a circle. Divide the chicken mix into 4 ramekins, top each with a dough circle, place in an oven at 375°F for 25 minutes. Serve the chicken pies warm.

Nutrition: Calories - 600, Fat - 54, Fiber - 14, Carbs - 10, Protein - 45

Bacon-wrapped Chicken

Preparation time: 10 minutes
Cooking time: 35 minutes
Servings: 4

Ingredients:
- 1 tablespoon fresh chives, chopped
- 8 ounces cream cheese
- 2 pounds chicken breasts, skinless and boneless
- 12 bacon slices
- Salt and ground black pepper, to taste

Directions:
Heat up a pan over medium heat, add the bacon, cook until halfway done, transfer to paper towels, and drain the grease. In a bowl, mix the cream cheese with salt, pepper, and chives, and stir. Use a meat tenderizer to flatten the chicken breasts well, add the cream cheese mixture, roll them up, and wrap each in a bacon slice. Arrange the wrapped chicken breasts into a baking dish, place in an oven at 375°F, and bake for 30 minutes.
Divide on plates and serve.

Nutrition: Calories - 700, Fat - 45, Fiber - 4, Carbs - 5, Protein - 45

Red-hot Chicken Wings

Preparation time: 10 minutes
Cooking time: 55 minutes
Servings: 4

Ingredients:
- 3 pounds chicken wings
- Salt and ground black pepper, to taste
- 3 tablespoons coconut aminos
- 2 teaspoons white vinegar
- 3 tablespoons rice vinegar
- 3 tablespoons stevia
- ¼ cup scallions, chopped
- ½ teaspoon xanthan gum
- 5 dried chilies, chopped

Directions:
Spread the chicken wings on a lined baking sheet, season with salt and pepper, place in an oven at 375°F, and bake for 45 minutes. Heat up a small pan over medium heat, add the white vinegar, rice vinegar, coconut aminos, stevia, xanthan gum, scallions, and chilies, stir well, bring to a boil, cook for 2 minutes, and take off the heat. Dip the chicken wings into this sauce, arrange them all on the baking sheet again, and bake for 10 minutes. Serve hot.

Nutrition: Calories - 415, Fat - 23, Fiber - 3, Carbs - 2, Protein - 27

Chicken in Creamy Sauce

Preparation time: 10 minutes
Cooking time: 1 hour and 10 minutes
Servings: 4

Ingredients:
- 8 chicken thighs
- Salt and ground black pepper, to taste
- 1 onion, peeled and chopped
- 1 tablespoon coconut oil
- 4 bacon strips, chopped
- 4 garlic cloves, peeled and minced
- 10 ounces cremini mushrooms, halved
- 2 cups chardonnay
- 1 cup whipping cream
- ½ cup fresh parsley, chopped

Directions:
Heat up a pan with the oil over medium heat, add the bacon, stir, cook until crispy, take off the heat, and transfer to paper towels. Heat up the pan with the bacon fat over medium heat, add the chicken pieces, season them with salt, and pepper, cook until brown, and transfer to paper towels. Heat up the pan again over medium heat, add the onions, stir, and cook for 6 minutes. Add the garlic, stir, cook for 1 minute, and transfer next to bacon pieces. Return the pan to stove and heat up again over medium temperature. Add the mushrooms, stir, and cook them for 5 minutes. Return the chicken, bacon, garlic, and onion to pan. Add the wine, stir, bring to a boil, reduce heat, and simmer for 40 minutes. Add the parsley and cream, stir, and cook for 10 minutes. Divide on plates and serve.

Nutrition: Calories - 340, Fat - 10, Fiber - 7, Carbs - 4, Protein - 24

Savory Chicken

Preparation time: 10 minutes
Cooking time: 1 hour
Servings: 4

Ingredients:
- 6 chicken breasts, skinless and boneless
- Salt and ground black pepper, to taste
- ¼ cup jalapeños, chopped
- 5 bacon slices, chopped
- 8 ounces cream cheese
- ¼ cup onion, peeled and chopped
- ½ cup mayonnaise
- ½ cup Parmesan cheese, grated
- 1 cup cheddar cheese, grated

For the topping:
- 2 ounces pork skins, crushed
- 4 tablespoons melted butter
- ½ cup Parmesan cheese

Directions:
Arrange the chicken breasts in a baking dish, season with salt, and pepper, place in an oven at 425ºF, and bake for 40 minutes. Heat up a pan over medium heat, add the bacon, stir, cook until crispy, and transfer to a plate. Heat up the pan again over medium heat, add the onions, stir, and cook for 4 minutes. Take off the heat, add the bacon, jalapeño, cream cheese, mayonnaise, cheddar cheese, and ½ cup Parmesan cheese, stir well, and spread over the chicken. In a bowl, mix the pork skin with butter, and ½ cup Parmesan cheese, and stir. Spread this over the chicken as well, place in an oven, and bake for 15 minutes. Serve hot.

Nutrition: Calories - 340, Fat - 12, Fiber - 2, Carbs - 5, Protein - 20

Chicken with Sour Cream Sauce

Preparation time: 10 minutes
Cooking time: 40 minutes
Servings: 4

Ingredients:
- 4 chicken thighs
- Salt and ground black pepper, to taste
- 1 teaspoon onion powder
- ¼ cup sour cream
- 2 tablespoons sweet paprika

Directions:
In a bowl, mix the paprika with salt, pepper, and onion powder, and stir. Season chicken pieces with this paprika mixture, arrange them on a lined baking sheet, and bake in the oven at 400ºF for 40 minutes. Divide the chicken on plates, and set aside. Pour the juices from the pan into a bowl, and add the sour cream. Stir this sauce well and drizzle over chicken.

Nutrition: Calories - 384, Fat - 31, Fiber - 2, Carbs - 1, Protein - 33

Chicken Stroganoff

Preparation time: 10 minutes
Cooking time: 4 hours and 10 minutes
Servings: 4

Ingredients:
- 2 garlic cloves, peeled and minced
- 8 ounces mushrooms, chopped
- ¼ teaspoon celery seeds, ground
- 1 cup chicken stock
- 1 cup coconut milk
- 1 onion, peeled and chopped
- 1 pound chicken breasts, cut into medium-sized pieces
- 1½ teaspoons dried thyme
- 2 tablespoons fresh parsley, chopped
- Salt and ground black pepper, to taste
- 4 zucchini, cut with a spiralizer

Directions:
Put the chicken in a slow cooker. Add the salt, pepper, onion, garlic, mushrooms, coconut milk, celery seeds, stock, half of the parsley, and thyme. Stir, cover, and cook on high for 4 hours. Uncover the pot, add more salt, and pepper, if needed, and the rest of the parsley, and stir. Heat up a pan with water over medium heat, add some salt, bring to a boil, add the zucchini pasta, cook for 1 minute, and drain. Divide on plates, add the chicken mixture on top, and serve.

Nutrition: Calories - 364, Fat - 22, Fiber - 2, Carbs - 4, Protein - 24

Chicken Gumbo

Preparation time: 10 minutes
Cooking time: 7 hours
Servings: 5

Ingredients:
- 2 sausages, sliced
- 3 chicken breasts, cubed
- 2 tablespoons dried oregano
- 2 bell peppers, seeded and chopped
- 1 onion, peeled and chopped
- 28 ounces canned diced tomatoes
- 3 tablespoons dried thyme
- 2 tablespoons garlic powder
- 2 tablespoons dry mustard
- 1 teaspoon cayenne powder
- 1 tablespoons chili powder
- Salt and ground black pepper, to taste
- 6 tablespoons Creole seasoning

Directions:
In a slow cooker, mix the sausages with the chicken, salt, pepper, bell peppers, oregano, onion, thyme, garlic powder, dry mustard, tomatoes, cayenne, chili, and Creole seasoning. Cover, and cook on low for 7 hours. Uncover the slow cooker again, stir the gumbo, and divide into bowls. Serve hot.

Nutrition: Calories - 360, Fat - 23, Fiber - 2, Carbs - 6, Protein - 23

Chicken Thighs with Mushrooms and Cheese

Preparation time: 10 minutes
Cooking time: 45 minutes
Servings: 4

Ingredients:
- 3 tablespoons butter
- 8 ounces mushrooms, sliced
- 2 tablespoons gruyere cheese, grated
- Salt and ground black pepper, to taste
- 2 garlic cloves, peeled and minced
- 6 chicken thighs

Directions:
Heat up a pan with 1 tablespoon butter over medium heat, add the chicken thighs, season with salt and pepper, cook for 3 minutes on each side, and arrange them in a baking dish. Heat up the pan again with the rest of the butter over medium heat, add the garlic, stir, and cook for 1 minute. Add the mushrooms and stir well. Add the salt and pepper, stir, and cook for 10 minutes. Spoon this mixture over the chicken, sprinkle with the cheese, place in an oven at 350°F, and bake for 30 minutes. Turn on the oven's broiler, and broil everything for a 2 minutes. Divide on plates and serve.

Nutrition: Calories - 340, Fat - 31, Fiber - 3, Carbs - 5, Protein - 64

Pecan-crusted Chicken

Preparation time: 10 minutes
Cooking time: 20 minutes
Servings: 4

Ingredients:
- 1 egg, whisked
- Salt and ground black pepper, to taste
- 3 tablespoons coconut oil
- 1½ cups pecans, chopped
- 4 chicken breasts
- Salt and ground black pepper, to taste

Directions:
Put the pecans in a bowl and the whisked egg in another. Season the chicken, dip in the egg and then in pecans. Heat up a pan with the oil over medium-high heat, add the chicken, and cook until brown on both sides. Transfer chicken pieces to a baking sheet, place in an oven, and bake at 350°F for 10 minutes. Divide on plates and serve.

Nutrition: Calories - 320, Fat - 12, Fiber - 4, Carbs - 1, Protein - 30

Pepperoni Chicken Bake

Preparation time: 10 minutes
Cooking time: 55 minutes
Servings: 6

Ingredients:
- 14 ounces low-carb pizza sauce
- 1 tablespoon coconut oil
- 4 medium chicken breasts, skinless and boneless
- Salt and ground black pepper, to taste
- 1 teaspoon dried oregano
- 6 ounces mozzarella cheese, sliced
- 1 teaspoon garlic powder
- 2 ounces pepperoni, sliced

Directions:
Put the pizza sauce in a small pot, bring to a boil over medium heat, simmer for 20 minutes, and take off the heat. In a bowl, mix the chicken with salt, pepper, garlic powder, and oregano, and stir. Heat up a pan with the coconut oil over medium-high heat, add the chicken pieces, cook for 2 minutes on each side, and transfer them to a baking dish. Add the mozzarella cheese slices on top, spread the sauce, top with the pepperoni slices, place in an oven at 400°F, and bake for 30 minutes. Divide on plates and serve.

Nutrition: Calories - 320, Fat - 10, Fiber - 6, Carbs - 3, Protein - 27

Fried Chicken

Preparation time: 24 hours
Cooking time: 20 minutes
Servings: 4

Ingredients:
- 3 chicken breasts, cut into strips
- 4 ounces pork rinds, crushed
- 2 cups coconut oil
- 16 ounces jarred pickle juice
- 2 eggs, whisked

Directions:
In a bowl, mix the chicken breast pieces with pickle juice, stir, cover, and keep in the refrigerator for 24 hours. Put the eggs in a bowl, and pork rinds in another one. Dip the chicken pieces in the egg, and then in pork rinds, and coat well. Heat up a pan with the oil over medium-high heat, add the chicken pieces, fry them for 3 minutes on each side, transfer them to paper towels, drain the grease, and serve.

Nutrition: Calories - 260, Fat - 5, Fiber - 1, Carbs - 2, Protein - 20

Chicken Calzone

Preparation time: 10 minutes
Cooking time: 1 hour
Servings: 12

Ingredients:
- 2 eggs
- 1 keto pizza crust
- ½ cup Parmesan cheese, grated
- 1 pound chicken breasts, skinless, boneless, and each sliced in half
- ½ cup keto marinara sauce
- 1 teaspoon Italian seasoning
- 1 teaspoon onion powder
- 1 teaspoon garlic powder
- Salt and ground black pepper, to taste
- ¼ cup flaxseed, ground
- 8 ounces provolone cheese

Directions:
In a bowl, mix the Italian seasoning with onion powder, garlic powder, salt, pepper, flaxseed, and Parmesan cheese, and stir well. In another bowl, mix the eggs with a pinch of salt, and pepper, and whisk. Dip the chicken pieces in eggs, and then in seasoning mixture, place all pieces on a lined baking sheet, and bake in the oven at 350°F for 30 minutes. Put the pizza crust dough on a lined baking sheet and spread half of the provolone cheese on half. Take the chicken out of the oven, chop it, and spread over the provolone cheese. Add the marinara sauce and then the rest of the cheese. Cover all these with the other half of the dough and shape the calzone. Seal the edges, place in an oven at 350°F, and bake for 20 minutes. Let the calzone to cool down before slicing and serving.

Nutrition: Calories - 340, Fat - 8, Fiber - 2, Carbs - 6, Protein - 20

Mexican Chicken Soup

Preparation time: 10 minutes
Cooking time: 4 hours
Servings: 6

Ingredients:
- 1½ pounds chicken tights, skinless, boneless, and cubed
- 15 ounces chicken stock
- 15 ounces canned chunky salsa
- 8 ounces Monterey jack

Directions:
In a slow cooker, mix the chicken with stock, salsa, and cheese, stir, cover, and cook on high for 4 hours. Uncover the slow cooker, stir the soup, divide into bowls, and serve.

Nutrition: Calories - 400, Fat - 22, Fiber - 3, Carbs - 6, Protein - 38

Simple Chicken Stir-fry

Preparation time: 10 minutes
Cooking time: 12 minutes
Servings: 2

Ingredients:
- 2 chicken thighs, skinless, boneless, and cut into thin strips
- 1 tablespoon sesame oil
- 1 teaspoon red pepper flakes
- 1 teaspoon onion powder
- 1 tablespoon fresh ginger, grated
- ¼ cup tamari sauce
- ½ teaspoon garlic powder
- ½ cup water
- 1 tablespoon stevia
- ½ teaspoon xanthan gum
- ½ cup scallions, chopped
- 2 cups broccoli florets

Directions:
Heat up a pan with the oil over medium-high heat, add the chicken and ginger, stir, and cook for 3 minutes. Add the water, tamari sauce, onion powder, garlic powder, stevia, pepper flakes, and xanthan gum, stir, and cook for 5 minutes. Add the broccoli and scallions, stir, cook for 2 minutes, and divide on plates. Serve hot.

Nutrition: Calories - 210, Fat - 10, Fiber - 3, Carbs - 5, Protein - 20

Spinach and Artichoke Chicken

Preparation time: 10 minutes
Cooking time: 50 minutes
Servings: 4

Ingredients:
- 4 ounces cream cheese
- 4 chicken breasts
- 10 ounces canned artichoke hearts, chopped
- 10 ounces spinach
- ½ cup Parmesan cheese, grated
- 1 tablespoon onion powder
- 1 tablespoon garlic powder
- Salt and ground black pepper, to taste
- 4 ounces mozzarella cheese, shredded

Directions:
Place the chicken breasts on a lined baking sheet, season with salt, and pepper, place in an oven at 400°F, and bake for 30 minutes. In a bowl, mix the artichokes with onion, cream cheese, Parmesan cheese, spinach, garlic, salt, and pepper, and stir. Take the chicken out of the oven, cut each piece in the middle, divide artichokes mixture, sprinkle with mozzarella cheese, place in an oven at 400°F, and bake for 15 minutes. Serve hot.

Nutrition: Calories - 450, Fat - 23, Fiber - 1, Carbs - 3, Protein - 39

Chicken Meatloaf

Preparation time: 10 minutes
Cooking time: 40 minutes
Servings: 8

Ingredients:
- 1 cup keto marinara sauce
- 2 pound ground chicken
- 2 tablespoons fresh parsley, chopped
- 4 garlic cloves, peeled and minced
- 2 teaspoons onion powder
- 2 teaspoons Italian seasoning
- Salt and ground black pepper, to taste

For the filling:
- ½ cup ricotta cheese
- 1 cup Parmesan cheese, grated
- 1 cup mozzarella cheese, shredded
- 2 teaspoons fresh chives, chopped
- 2 tablespoons fresh parsley, chopped
- 1 garlic clove, peeled and minced

Directions:
In a bowl, mix the chicken with half of the marinara sauce, salt, pepper, Italian seasoning, 4 garlic cloves, onion powder, and 2 tablespoons parsley, and stir well. In another bowl, mix the ricotta cheese with half of the Parmesan cheese, half of the mozzarella cheese, chives, 1 garlic clove, salt, pepper, and 2 tablespoons parsley, and stir well. Put half of the chicken mix into a loaf pan, and spread evenly. Add the cheese filling and spread evenly. Top with the rest of the meat and spread again. Place the meatloaf in the oven at 400°F and bake for 20 minutes. Take the meatloaf out of the oven, spread the rest of the marinara sauce, the rest of the cheese, and bake for 20 minutes. Let the meatloaf to cool down, slice, divide on plates, and serve.

Nutrition: Calories - 273, Fat - 14, Fiber - 1, Carbs - 4, Protein - 28

One-pot Roasted Chicken

Preparation time: 10 minutes
Cooking time: 40 minutes
Servings: 12

Ingredients:
- 1 whole chicken
- ½ teaspoon onion powder
- ½ teaspoon garlic powder
- Salt and ground black pepper, to taste
- 2 tablespoons coconut oil
- 1 teaspoon Italian seasoning
- 1½ cups chicken stock
- 2 teaspoons guar gum

Directions:
Rub the chicken with half of the oil, garlic powder, salt, pepper, Italian seasoning, and onion powder. Put the rest of the oil into an Instant Pot, and add chicken to the pot. Add the stock, cover the Instant Pot, and cook on Poultry mode for 40 minutes. Transfer the chicken to a platter, and set aside. Set the instant pot on Sauté mode, add the guar gum, stir, and cook until it thickens. Pour sauce over chicken and serve.

Nutrition: Calories - 450, Fat - 30, Fiber - 1, Carbs - 1, Protein - 34

Chicken with Green Onion Sauce

Preparation time: 10 minutes
Cooking time: 27 minutes
Servings: 4

Ingredients:
- 2 tablespoons butter
- 1 green onion, peeled and chopped
- 4 chicken breast halves, skinless and boneless
- Salt and ground black pepper, to taste
- 8 ounces sour cream

Directions:
Heat up a pan with the butter over medium-high heat, add the chicken pieces, season with salt and pepper, cover, reduce heat, and simmer for 10 minutes. Uncover the pan, turn the chicken pieces, and cook them covered for 10 minutes. Add the green onions, stir, and cook for 2 minutes. Take off the heat, add more salt, and pepper if needed, add the sour cream, stir well, cover the pan, and set aside for 5 minutes. Stir again, divide on plates, and serve.

Nutrition: Calories - 200, Fat - 7, Fiber - 2, Carbs - 1, Protein - 8

Chicken-stuffed Mushrooms

Preparation time: 10 minutes
Cooking time: 10 minutes
Servings: 6

Ingredients:
- 16 ounces button mushroom caps
- 4 ounces cream cheese
- ¼ cup carrot, chopped
- 1 teaspoon ranch seasoning mix
- 4 tablespoons hot sauce
- ¾ cup blue cheese, crumbled
- ¼ cup onion, chopped
- ½ cup chicken meat, already cooked and chopped
- Salt and ground black pepper, to taste
- Vegetable oil cooking spray

Directions:
In a bowl, mix the cream cheese with the blue cheese, hot sauce, ranch seasoning, salt, pepper, chicken, carrot, and onion, and stir. Stuff each mushroom cap with this mixture, place them all on a lined baking sheet, spray with cooking spray, place in an oven at 425°F, and bake for 10 minutes. Divide on plates and serve.

Nutrition: Calories - 200, Fat - 4, Fiber - 1, Carbs - 2, Protein - 7

Chicken-stuffed Avocados

Preparation time: 10 minutes
Cooking time: 0 minutes
Servings: 2

Ingredients:
- 2 avocados, cut in half and pitted
- ¼ cup mayonnaise
- 1 teaspoon dried thyme
- 2 tablespoons cream cheese
- 1½ cups chicken, cooked and shredded
- Salt and ground black pepper, to taste
- ¼ teaspoon cayenne pepper
- ½ teaspoon onion powder
- ½ teaspoon garlic powder
- 1 teaspoon paprika
- Salt and ground black pepper, to taste
- 2 tablespoons lemon juice

Directions:
Scoop the insides of the avocado halves, and put the flesh in a bowl. Let the avocado cups aside for now. Add the chicken to the avocado flesh and stir. Add the mayonnaise, thyme, cream cheese, cayenne, onion, garlic, paprika, salt, pepper, and lemon juice, and stir well. Stuff avocados with chicken mixture and serve.

Nutrition: Calories - 230, Fat - 40, Fiber - 11, Carbs - 5, Protein - 24

Balsamic Chicken

Preparation time: 10 minutes
Cooking time: 20 minutes
Servings: 4

Ingredients:
- 3 tablespoons coconut oil
- 2 pounds chicken breasts, skinless and boneless
- 3 garlic cloves, peeled and minced
- Salt and ground black pepper, to taste
- 1 cup chicken stock
- 3 tablespoons stevia
- ½ cup balsamic vinegar
- 1 tomato, sliced thin
- 6 mozzarella slices
- Fresh basil, chopped, for serving

Directions:
Heat up a pan with the oil over medium-high heat, add the chicken pieces, season with salt and pepper, cook until brown on both sides, and reduce heat. Add the garlic, vinegar, stock, and stevia, stir, increase heat again, and cook for 10 minutes. Transfer the chicken breasts to a lined baking sheet, arrange mozzarella cheese slices on top, and then top with the basil. Broil in the oven over medium heat until cheese melts and arrange tomato slices over chicken pieces. Divide on plates and serve.

Nutrition: Calories - 240, Fat - 12, Fiber - 1, Carbs - 4, Protein - 27

Chicken Pasta

Preparation time: 10 minutes
Cooking time: 30 minutes
Servings: 4

Ingredients:
- 2 tablespoons butter
- 1 teaspoon garlic, minced
- 1 pound chicken cutlets
- 1 teaspoon Cajun seasoning
- ¼ cup scallions, chopped
- ½ cup tomatoes, cored and chopped
- ½ cup chicken stock
- ¼ cup whipping cream
- ½ cup cheddar cheese, grated
- 1 ounce cream cheese
- ¼ cup fresh cilantro, chopped
- Salt and ground black pepper, to taste

For the pasta:
- 4 ounces cream cheese
- 8 eggs
- Salt and ground black pepper, to taste
- A pinch of garlic powder

Directions:
Heat up a pan with 1 tablespoon butter over medium heat, add the chicken cutlets, season with some of the Cajun seasoning, cook for 2 minutes on each side, and transfer to a plate. Heat up the pan with the rest of the butter over medium heat, add the garlic, stir, and cook for 2 minutes. Add the tomatoes, stir, and cook for 2 minutes. Add the stock and the rest of the Cajun seasoning, stir, and cook for 5 minutes. Add the whipping cream, cheddar cheese, 1 ounce cream cheese, salt, pepper, scallions, and cilantro, stir well, cook for 2 minutes, and take off the heat. In a blender, mix the 4 ounces cream cheese with eggs, salt, pepper, and garlic powder, and pulse well. Pour this into a lined baking sheet, set aside for 5 minutes, and then bake in the oven at 325°F for 10 minutes. Let the pasta sheet to cool down, transfer to a cutting board, roll, and cut into medium slices. Divide pasta on plates, top with chicken mixture, and serve.

Nutrition: Calories - 345, Fat - 34, Fiber - 4, Carbs - 4, Protein - 39

Peanut-grilled Chicken

Preparation time: 10 minutes
Cooking time: 20 minutes
Servings: 8

Ingredients:
- 2½ pounds chicken thighs, and drumsticks
- 1 tablespoon coconut aminos
- 1 tablespoon apple cider vinegar
- A pinch of red pepper flakes
- Salt and ground black pepper, to taste
- ½ teaspoon ground ginger
- ⅓ cup peanut butter
- 1 garlic clove, peeled and minced
- ½ cup warm water

Directions:
In a blender, mix the peanut butter with water, aminos, salt, pepper, pepper flakes, ginger, garlic, and vinegar, and blend well. Pat the chicken pieces dry, arrange them in a pan, and pour the peanut butter marinade over it. Toss to coat and keep in the refrigerator for 1 hour. Place the chicken pieces skin side down on a preheated grill over medium-high heat, cook for 10 minutes, flip, brush with some of the marinade, and cook them for 10 minutes. Divide on plates and serve.

Nutrition: Calories - 375, Fat - 12, Fiber - 1, Carbs - 3, Protein - 42

Chicken Stew

Preparation time: 10 minutes
Cooking time: 2 hours
Servings: 4

Ingredients:
- 2 carrots, peeled and chopped
- 2 celery stalks, chopped
- 2 cups chicken stock
- 1 small onion, peeled and chopped
- 28 ounces chicken thighs, skinless, boneless, and cut into medium-sized pieces
- 3 garlic cloves, peeled and minced
- ½ teaspoon dried rosemary
- 1 cup spinach
- ½ teaspoon dried oregano
- ¼ teaspoon dried thyme
- ½ cup heavy cream
- Salt and ground black pepper, to taste
- A pinch of xanthan gum

Directions:
In a slow cooker, mix the chicken with the stock, celery, carrots, onion, garlic, rosemary, thyme, oregano, some salt, and pepper, stir, cover, and cook on high for 2 hours. Add more salt and pepper, spinach, and heavy cream, and stir. Add the xanthan gum, stir, and cook for 10 minutes. Divide into bowls and serve.

Nutrition: Calories - 224, Fat - 11, Fiber - 4, Carbs - 6, Protein - 23

Chicken and Vegetable Stew

Preparation time: 10 minutes
Cooking time: 30 minutes
Servings: 6

Ingredients:
- 2 cups whipping cream
- 40 ounces rotisserie chicken pieces, boneless, skinless, and shredded
- 3 tablespoons butter
- ½ cup onion, chopped
- ¾ cup red bell pepper, chopped
- 29 ounces canned chicken stock
- Salt and ground black pepper, to taste
- 1 bay leaf
- 8 ounces mushrooms, chopped
- 1 cup green snap beans
- 17 ounces asparagus, trimmed
- 3 teaspoons fresh thyme, chopped

Directions:
Heat up a pan with the cream over medium heat, bring to a simmer, and cook until it's reduced to 7 minutes.
Heat up a pan with the butter over medium heat, add the onion and peppers, stir, and cook for 3 minutes. Add the stock, bay leaf, and some salt and pepper, bring to a boil, and simmer for 10 minutes. Add the asparagus, green beans, and mushrooms, stir, and cook for 7 minutes. Add the chicken pieces, stir, and cook for 3 minutes. Add the cream, thyme, and salt and pepper to taste, stir, discard the bay leaf, divide stew into bowls, and serve.

Nutrition: Calories - 500, Fat - 27, Fiber - 3, Carbs - 4, Protein - 47

Ketogenic Meat Recipes

Roasted Pork Belly

Preparation time: 10 minutes
Cooking time: 1 hour and 30 minutes
Servings: 6

Ingredients:
- 2 tablespoons stevia
- 1 tablespoon lemon juice
- 1 quart water
- 17 ounces apples, cored, and cut into wedges
- 2 pounds pork belly, scored
- Salt and ground black pepper, to taste
- A drizzle of olive oil

Directions:
In a blender, mix the water with apples, lemon juice, and stevia, and pulse well. Put the pork belly in a steamer tray and steam for 1 hour. Transfer the pork belly to a baking sheet, rub with a drizzle of oil, season with salt and pepper, and pour the apple sauce over it. Place in an oven at 425ºF for 30 minutes. Slice the pork roast, divide on plates, and serve with the applesauce on top.

Nutrition: Calories - 456, Fat - 34, Fiber - 4, Carbs - 10, Protein - 25

Stuffed Pork

Preparation time: 10 minutes
Cooking time: 30 minutes
Servings: 4

Ingredients:
- Zest of 2 limes
- Zest from 1 orange
- Juice from 1 orange
- Juice from 2 limes
- 4 teaspoons garlic, peeled, and minced
- ¾ cup olive oil
- 1 cup fresh cilantro, chopped
- 1 cup fresh mint, chopped
- 1 teaspoon dried oregano
- Salt and ground black pepper, to taste
- 2 teaspoons cumin
- 4 pork loin steaks
- 2 pickles, chopped
- 4 ham slices
- 6 Swiss cheese slices
- 2 tablespoons mustard

Directions:
In a food processor, mix the lime zest, lime juice, orange zest, orange juice, garlic, oil, cilantro, mint, oregano, cumin, salt, and pepper, and blend well. Season the steaks with salt and pepper, place them into a bowl, add the marinade, toss to coat, and set aside for a couple of hours. Place the steaks on a working surface, divide the pickles, cheese, mustard, and ham on them, roll, and secure with toothpicks. Heat up a pan over medium-high heat, add the pork rolls, cook them for 2 minutes on each side, and transfer them to a baking sheet. Place in an oven at 350ºF, and bake for 25 minutes. Divide on plates and serve.

Nutrition: Calories - 270, Fat - 7, Fiber - 2, Carbs - 3, Protein - 20

Pork Chops with Mushrooms

Preparation time: 10 minutes
Cooking time: 40 minutes
Servings: 3

Ingredients:
- 8 ounces mushrooms, sliced
- 1 teaspoon garlic powder
- 1 onion, peeled and chopped
- 1 cup mayonnaise
- 3 pork chops, boneless
- 1 teaspoon ground nutmeg
- 1 tablespoon balsamic vinegar
- ½ cup coconut oil

Directions:
Heat up a pan with the oil over medium heat, add the mushrooms and onions, stir, and cook for 4 minutes. Add the pork chops, season with nutmeg, and garlic powder, and brown on both sides. Place the pan in the oven at 350°F, and bake for 30 minutes. Transfer pork chops to plates and keep warm. Heat up the pan over medium heat, add the vinegar, and mayonnaise over the mushrooms mixture, stir well, and take off the heat. Drizzle sauce over pork chops and serve.

Nutrition: Calories - 600, Fat - 10, Fiber - 1, Carbs - 8, Protein - 30

Italian Pork Rolls

Preparation time: 10 minutes
Cooking time: 20 minutes
Servings: 6

Ingredients:
- 6 prosciutto slices
- 2 tablespoons fresh parsley, chopped
- 1 pound pork cutlets, sliced thin
- ⅓ cup ricotta cheese
- 1 tablespoon coconut oil
- ¼ cup onion, chopped
- 3 garlic cloves, peeled and minced
- 2 tablespoons Parmesan cheese, grated
- 15 ounces canned diced tomatoes
- ⅓ cup chicken stock
- Salt and ground black pepper, to taste
- ½ teaspoon Italian seasoning

Directions:
Use a meat pounder to flatten the pork pieces. Place the prosciutto slices on top of each piece, then divide the ricotta cheese, parsley, and Parmesan cheese. Roll each pork piece and secure with a toothpick. Heat up a pan with the oil over medium heat, add the pork rolls, cook until they are brown on both sides, and transfer to a plate. Heat up the pan again over medium heat, add the garlic and onion, stir, and cook for 5 minutes. Add the stock and cook for 3 minutes. Discard the toothpicks from pork rolls and return them to the pan. Add the tomatoes, Italian seasoning, salt, and pepper, stir, bring to a boil, reduce heat to medium-low, cover pan, and cook for 30 minutes. Divide on plates and serve.

Nutrition: Calories - 280, Fat - 17, Fiber - 1, Carbs - 2, Protein - 34

Lemon and Garlic Pork

Preparation time: 10 minutes
Cooking time: 30 minutes
Servings: 4

Ingredients:
- 3 tablespoons butter
- 4 pork steaks, bone-in
- 1 cup chicken stock
- Salt and ground black pepper, to taste
- A pinch of lemon pepper
- 3 tablespoons coconut oil
- 6 garlic cloves, peeled and minced
- 2 tablespoons fresh parsley, chopped
- 8 ounces mushrooms, chopped
- 1 lemon, sliced

Directions:
Heat up a pan with 2 tablespoons butter and 2 tablespoons oil over medium-high heat, add the pork steaks, season with salt and pepper, cook until they are brown on both sides, and transfer to a plate. Return the pan to medium heat, add the rest of the butter, and oil, and half of the stock. Stir well, and cook for 1 minute. Add the mushrooms and garlic, stir, and cook for 4 minutes. Add the lemon slices, the rest of the stock, salt, pepper, and lemon pepper, stir, and cook everything for 5 minutes. Return the pork steaks to pan and cook everything for 10 minutes. Divide the steaks and sauce on plates and serve.

Nutrition: Calories - 456, Fat - 25, Fiber - 1, Carbs - 6, Protein - 40

Jamaican Pork

Preparation time: 10 minutes
Cooking time: 45 minutes
Servings: 12

Ingredients:
- 4 pounds pork shoulder
- 1 tablespoon coconut oil
- ½ cup beef stock
- ¼ cup Jamaican jerk spice mix

Directions:
Rub the pork shoulder with Jamaican mixture, and place in an Instant Pot. Add the oil to the pot, and set it to Sauté mode. Add the pork shoulder, and brown it on all sides. Add the stock, cover the Instant Pot, and cook on Meat/Stew mode for 45 minutes. Uncover the Instant Pot, transfer pork to a platter, shred, and serve.

Nutrition: Calories - 267, Fat - 20, Fiber - 0, Carbs - 0, Protein - 24

Cranberry Pork Roast

Preparation time: 10 minutes
Cooking time: 8 hours
Servings: 4

Ingredients:
- 1 tablespoon coconut flour
- Salt and ground black pepper, to taste
- 1½ pounds pork loin
- A pinch of dry mustard
- ½ teaspoon ginger
- 2 tablespoons sugar substitute
- 2 tablespoons brown sugar substitute
- ½ cup cranberries
- 2 garlic cloves, peeled and minced
- ½ lemon sliced
- ¼ cup water

Directions:
In a bowl, mix the ginger with the mustard, salt, pepper, and flour, and stir. Add the roast, toss to coat, and transfer meat to a slow cooker. Add the sugar substitute, brown sugar substitute, cranberries, garlic, water, and lemon slices. Cover the slow cooker and cook on low for 8 hours. Divide on plates, drizzle pan juices on top, and serve.

Nutrition: Calories - 430, Fat - 23, Fiber - 2, Carbs - 3, Protein - 45

Juicy Pork Chops

Preparation time: 10 minutes
Cooking time: 45 minutes
Servings: 4

Ingredients:
- 2 onions, peeled and chopped
- 6 bacon slices, chopped
- ½ cup chicken stock
- Salt and ground black pepper, to taste
- 4 pork chops

Directions:
Heat up a pan over medium heat, add the bacon, stir, cook until crispy, and transfer to a bowl. Return the pan to medium heat, add the onions and some salt and pepper, stir, cover, cook for 15 minutes, and transfer to the same bowl with the bacon. Return this to the heat, increase to medium-high, add the pork chops, season with salt and pepper, brown for 3 minutes on one side, flip, reduce heat to medium, and cook for 7 minutes. Add the stock, stir, and cook for 2 minutes. Return the bacon and onions to the pan, stir, cook for 1 minute, divide on plates, and serve.

Nutrition: Calories - 325, Fat - 18, Fiber - 1, Carbs - 6, Protein - 36

Lemon Pork Chops

Preparation time: 10 minutes
Cooking time: 15 minutes
Servings: 4

Ingredients:
- 4 medium pork loin chops
- 1 teaspoon Dijon mustard
- 1 tablespoon Worcestershire sauce
- 1 teaspoon lemon juice
- 1 tablespoon water
- Salt and ground black pepper, to taste
- 1 teaspoon lemon pepper
- 1 tablespoon butter
- 1 tablespoon fresh chives, chopped

Directions:
In a bowl, mix the water with Worcestershire sauce, mustard, and lemon juice, and whisk. Heat up a pan with the butter over medium heat, add the pork chops, season with salt, pepper, and lemon pepper, cook them for 6 minutes, flip, and cook for 6 more minutes. Transfer the pork chops to a platter and keep warm.
Heat up the pan again, add the mustard sauce, and bring to a gentle simmer. Pour this over pork, sprinkle with chives, and serve.

Nutrition: Calories - 132, Fat - 5, Fiber - 1, Carbs - 1, Protein - 18

Mediterranean Pork

Preparation time: 10 minutes
Cooking time: 35 minutes
Servings: 4

Ingredients:
- 4 pork chops, bone-in
- Salt and ground black pepper, to taste
- 1 teaspoon dried rosemary
- 3 garlic cloves, peeled and minced

Directions:
Season the pork chops with salt and pepper, and place in a roasting pan. Add the rosemary and garlic, place in an oven at 425°F, and bake for 10 minutes. Reduce heat to 350°F and roast for 25 minutes. Slice the pork, divide on plates, and drizzle with pan juices all over.

Nutrition: Calories - 165, Fat - 2, Fiber - 1, Carbs - 2, Protein - 26

Italian Pork Chops

Preparation time: 10 minutes
Cooking time: 40 minutes
Servings: 4

Ingredients:
- 4 pork chops
- 1 tablespoon fresh oregano, chopped
- 2 garlic cloves, peeled and minced
- 1 tablespoon canola oil
- 15 ounces canned diced tomatoes
- 1 tablespoon tomato paste
- Salt and ground black pepper, to taste
- ¼ cup tomato juice

Directions:
Heat up a pan with the oil over medium-high heat, add the pork chops, season with salt and pepper, cook for 3 minutes, flip, cook for 3 minutes, and transfer to a plate. Return the pan to medium heat, add the garlic, stir, and cook for 10 seconds. Add the tomato juice, tomatoes, and tomato paste, stir, bring to a boil, and reduce heat to medium-low. Add the pork chops, stir, cover pan, and simmer everything for 30 minutes. Transfer the pork chops to plates, add the oregano to the pan, stir, and cook for 2 minutes. Pour this over the pork and serve.

Nutrition: Calories - 210, Fat - 10, Fiber - 2, Carbs - 6, Protein - 19

Spicy Pork Chops

Preparation time: 4 hours and 10 minutes
Cooking time: 15 minutes
Servings: 4

Ingredients:
- ¼ cup lime juice
- 4 pork rib chops
- 1 tablespoon coconut oil, melted
- 2 garlic cloves, peeled and minced
- 1 tablespoon chili powder
- 1 teaspoon ground cinnamon
- 2 teaspoons cumin
- Salt and ground black pepper, to taste
- ½ teaspoon hot pepper sauce
- Sliced mango, for serving

Directions:
In a bowl, mix the lime juice with oil, garlic, cumin, cinnamon, chili powder, salt, pepper, and hot pepper sauce, and whisk. Add the pork chops, toss to coat, and set aside in the refrigerator for 4 hours. Place the pork on a preheated grill over medium heat, cook for 7 minutes, flip, and cook for 7 minutes. Divide on plates and serve with mango slices on the side.

Nutrition: Calories - 200, Fat - 8, Fiber - 1, Carbs - 3, Protein - 26

Thai Beef

Preparation time: 10 minutes
Cooking time: 10 minutes
Servings: 6

Ingredients:
- 1 cup beef stock
- 4 tablespoons peanut butter
- ¼ teaspoon garlic powder
- ¼ teaspoon onion powder
- 1 tablespoon coconut aminos
- 1½ teaspoons lemon pepper
- 1 pound beef steak, cut into strips
- Salt and ground black pepper, to taste
- 1 green bell pepper, seeded and chopped
- 3 green onions, chopped

Directions:
In a bowl, mix the peanut butter with the stock, aminos, and lemon pepper, stir well, and set aside. Heat up a pan over medium-high heat, add the beef, season with salt, pepper, onion, and garlic powder, and cook for 7 minutes. Add the green pepper, stir, and cook for 3 minutes. Add the peanut sauce and green onions, stir, cook for 1 minute, divide on plates, and serve.

Nutrition: Calories - 224, Fat - 15, Fiber - 1, Carbs - 3, Protein - 19

Beef Patties

Preparation time: 10 minutes
Cooking time: 35 minutes
Servings: 6

Ingredients:
- ½ cup bread crumbs
- 1 egg
- Salt and ground black pepper, to taste
- 1½ pounds ground beef
- 10 ounces canned onion soup
- 1 tablespoon coconut flour
- ¼ cup ketchup
- 3 teaspoons Worcestershire sauce
- ½ teaspoon dry mustard
- ¼ cup water

Directions:
In a bowl, mix ⅓ cup of the onion soup with the beef, salt, pepper, egg, and bread crumbs, and stir well. Heat up a pan over medium-high heat, shape 6 patties from the beef mixture, place them into the pan, and brown on both sides. In a bowl, mix the rest of the soup with the coconut flour, water, dry mustard, Worcestershire sauce, and ketchup, and stir well. Pour this over the beef patties, cover pan, and cook for 20 minutes stirring from time to time. Divide on plates and serve.

Nutrition: Calories - 332, Fat - 18, Fiber - 1, Carbs - 7, Protein - 25

Beef Pot Roast

Preparation time: 10 minutes
Cooking time: 1 hour and 15 minutes
Servings: 4

Ingredients:
- 3½ pounds beef roast
- 4 ounces mushrooms, sliced
- 12 ounces beef stock
- 1 ounce onion soup mix
- ½ cup Italian dressing

Directions:
In a bowl, mix the stock with the onion soup mixture and Italian dressing, and stir. Put the beef roast in a pan, add the mushrooms, stock mixture, cover with aluminum foil, place in an oven at 300ºF, and bake for 1 hour and 15 minutes. Let the roast to cool, slice, and serve with the gravy on top.

Nutrition: Calories - 700, Fat - 56, Fiber - 2, Carbs - 10, Protein - 70

Beef Zucchini Cups

Preparation time: 10 minutes
Cooking time: 35 minutes
Servings: 4

Ingredients:
- 2 garlic cloves, peeled and minced
- 1 teaspoon cumin
- 1 tablespoon coconut oil
- 1 pound ground beef
- ½ cup onion, chopped
- 1 teaspoon smoked paprika
- Salt and ground black pepper, to taste
- 3 zucchini, sliced in half lengthwise, and insides scooped out
- ¼ cup fresh cilantro, chopped
- ½ cup cheddar cheese, shredded
- 1½ cups keto enchilada sauce
- Avocado, chopped, for serving
- Green onions, chopped, for serving
- Tomatoes, cored, and chopped, for serving

Directions:
Heat up a pan with the oil over medium-high heat, add the onions, stir, and cook for 2 minutes. Add the beef, stir, and brown for a couple of minutes. Add the paprika, salt, pepper, cumin, and garlic, stir, and cook for 2 minutes. Place the zucchini halves in a baking pan, stuff each with the beef, pour the enchilada sauce on top, and sprinkle with the cheddar cheese. Bake covered in the oven at 350ºF for 20 minutes. Uncover the pan, sprinkle with the cilantro, and bake for 5 minutes. Sprinkle with the avocado, green onions, and tomatoes on top, divide on plates, and serve.

Nutrition: Calories - 222, Fat - 10, Fiber - 2, Carbs - 8, Protein - 21

Beef Meatball Casserole

Preparation time: 10 minutes
Cooking time: 50 minutes
Servings: 8

Ingredients:
- ⅓ cup almond flour
- 2 eggs
- 1 pound beef sausage, chopped
- 1 pound ground beef
- Salt and ground black pepper, to taste to taste
- 1 tablespoons dried parsley
- ¼ teaspoon red pepper flakes
- ¼ cup Parmesan cheese, grated
- ¼ teaspoon onion powder
- ½ teaspoon garlic powder
- ¼ teaspoon dried oregano
- 1 cup ricotta cheese
- 2 cups keto marinara sauce
- 1½ cups mozzarella cheese, shredded

Directions:
In a bowl, mix the sausage with the beef, salt, pepper, almond flour, parsley, pepper flakes, onion powder, garlic powder, oregano, Parmesan cheese, and eggs, and stir well. Shape the meatballs, place them on a lined baking sheet, place in an oven at 375°F, and bake for 15 minutes. Take the meatballs out of the oven, transfer them to a baking dish, and cover with half of the marinara sauce. Add the ricotta cheese all over and then pour the rest of the marinara sauce. Sprinkle the mozzarella cheese all over, place the dish in the oven at 375°F, and bake for 30 minutes. Let the meatballs casserole to cool before cutting and serving.

Nutrition: Calories - 456, Fat - 35, Fiber - 3, Carbs - 4, Protein - 32

Beef and Tomato-stuffed Squash

Preparation time: 10 minutes
Cooking time: 1 hour
Servings: 2

Ingredients:
- 2 pounds acorn squash, pricked with a fork
- Salt and ground black pepper, to taste
- 3 garlic cloves, peeled and minced
- 1 onion, peeled and chopped
- 1 Portobello mushroom, sliced
- 28 ounces canned diced tomatoes
- 1 teaspoon dried oregano
- ¼ teaspoon cayenne pepper
- ½ teaspoon dried thyme
- 1 pound ground beef
- 1 green bell pepper, seeded and chopped

Directions:
Place the acorn squash on a lined baking sheet, place in an oven at 400°F, and bake for 40 minutes. Cut in half, set aside to cool down, remove seeds, and leave aside. Heat up a pan over medium-high heat, add the meat, garlic, onion, and mushroom, stir, and cook until the meat browns. Add the salt, pepper, thyme, oregano, cayenne, tomatoes, and green pepper, stir, and cook for 10 minutes. Stuff the squash halves with the beef mixture, place in an oven at 400°F, and bake for 10 minutes. Divide between 2 plates and serve.

Nutrition: Calories - 260, Fat - 7, Fiber - 2, Carbs - 4, Protein - 10

Beef Chili

Preparation time: 10 minutes
Cooking time: 8 hours
Servings: 4

Ingredients:
- 1 onion, peeled and chopped
- 2½ pounds ground beef
- 15 ounces canned tomatoes, and green chilies, chopped
- 6 ounces tomato paste
- ½ cup pickled jalapeños, chopped
- 4 tablespoons garlic, minced
- 3 celery stalks, chopped
- 2 tablespoons coconut aminos
- 4 tablespoons chili powder
- Salt and ground black pepper, to taste
- A pinch of cayenne pepper
- 2 tablespoons cumin
- 1 teaspoon onion powder
- 1 teaspoon garlic powder
- 1 bay leaf
- 1 teaspoon dried oregano

Directions:
Heat up a pan over medium-high heat, add the half of the onion, beef, half of the garlic, salt, and pepper, stir, and cook until meat browns. Transfer this to a slow cooker, add the rest of the onion and garlic, plus the jalapeños, celery, tomatoes, chilies, tomato paste, canned tomatoes, coconut aminos, chili powder, salt, pepper, cumin, garlic powder, onion powder, oregano, and bay leaf, stir, cover, and cook on low for 8 hours. Divide into bowls and serve.

Nutrition: Calories - 137, Fat - 6, Fiber - 2, Carbs - 5, Protein - 17

Glazed Beef Meatloaf

Preparation time: 10 minutes
Cooking time: 1 hour and 10 minutes
Servings: 6

Ingredients:
- 1 cup white mushrooms, chopped
- 3 pounds ground beef
- 2 tablespoons fresh parsley, chopped
- 2 garlic cloves, peeled and minced
- ½ cup onion, chopped
- ¼ cup red bell pepper, seeded and chopped
- ½ cup almond flour
- ⅓ cup Parmesan cheese, grated
- 3 eggs
- Salt and ground black pepper, to taste
- 1 teaspoon balsamic vinegar

For the glaze:
- 1 tablespoon swerve
- 2 tablespoons sugar-free ketchup
- 2 cups balsamic vinegar

Directions:
In a bowl, mix the beef with salt, pepper, mushrooms, garlic, onion, bell pepper, parsley, almond flour, Parmesan cheese, 1 teaspoon vinegar, salt, pepper, and eggs, and stir well. Transfer this into a loaf pan, and bake in the oven at 375°F for 30 minutes. Heat up a small pan over medium heat, add the ketchup, swerve, and 2 cups vinegar, stir well, and cook for 20 minutes. Take the meatloaf out of the oven, spread the glaze over the meatloaf, place in an oven at the same temperature, and bake for 20 minutes. Let the meatloaf cool, slice, and serve it.

Nutrition: Calories - 264, Fat - 14, Fiber - 3, Carbs - 5, Protein - 24

Beef with Tzatziki

Preparation time: 10 minutes
Cooking time: 15 minutes
Servings: 6

Ingredients:
- ¼ cup almond milk
- 17 ounces ground beef
- 1 onion, peeled, and grated
- 5 bread slices, torn
- 1 egg, whisked
- ¼ cup fresh parsley, chopped
- Salt and ground black pepper, to taste
- 2 garlic cloves, peeled and minced
- ¼ cup fresh mint, chopped
- 2, and ½ teaspoons dried oregano
- ¼ cup olive oil
- 7 ounces cherry tomatoes, cut in half
- 1 cucumber, sliced thin
- 1 cup baby spinach
- 1½ tablespoons lemon juice
- 7 ounces jarred tzatziki

Directions:
Put the torn bread in a bowl, add the milk, and set aside for 3 minutes. Squeeze the bread, chop, and put into a bowl. Add the beef, egg, salt, pepper, oregano, mint, parsley, garlic, and onion, and stir well. Shape balls from this mixture and place on a working surface. Heat up a pan with half of the oil over medium-high heat, add the meatballs, cook them for 8 minutes flipping them from time to time, and transfer them all to a tray. In a salad bowl, mix the spinach with the cucumber and tomato. Add the meatballs, the rest of the oil, and some salt, pepper, and lemon juice. Add tzatziki, toss to coat, and serve.

Nutrition: Calories - 200, Fat - 4, Fiber - 1, Carbs - 3, Protein - 7

Meatballs with Mushroom Sauce

Preparation time: 10 minutes
Cooking time: 25 minutes
Servings: 6

Ingredients:
- 2 pounds ground beef
- Salt and ground black pepper, to taste
- ½ teaspoon garlic powder
- 1 tablespoon coconut aminos
- ¼ cup beef stock
- ¾ cup almond flour
- 1 tablespoon fresh parsley, chopped
- 1 tablespoon dried onion flakes
- 1 cup onion, chopped
- 2 cups mushrooms, sliced
- 2 tablespoons bacon fat
- 2 tablespoons butter
- ½ teaspoon coconut aminos
- ¼ cup sour cream
- ½ cup beef stock
- Salt and ground black pepper, to taste

For the sauce:

Directions:
In a bowl, mix the beef with salt, pepper, garlic powder, 1 tablespoons coconut aminos, ¼ cup beef stock, almond flour, parsley, and onion flakes, stir well, shape 6 patties, place them on a baking sheet, place in an oven at 375°F, and bake for 18 minutes. Heat up a pan with the butter, and the bacon fat over medium heat, add the mushrooms, stir, and cook for 4 minutes. Add the onions, stir, and cook for 4 minutes. Add the ½ teaspoon coconut aminos, sour cream, and ½ cup beef stock, stir well, and bring to a simmer. Take off heat, add the salt, and pepper, and stir well. Divide the beef patties on plates, and serve with mushroom sauce on top.

Nutrition: Calories - 435, Fat - 23, Fiber - 4, Carbs - 6, Protein - 32

Beef and Sauerkraut Soup

Preparation time: 10 minutes
Cooking time: 1 hour and 20 minutes
Servings: 8

Ingredients:
- 3 teaspoons olive oil
- 1 pound ground beef
- 14 ounces beef stock
- 2 cups chicken stock
- 14 ounces canned tomatoes, and juice
- 1 tablespoon stevia
- 14 ounces sauerkraut, chopped
- 1 tablespoon gluten-free Worcestershire sauce
- 4 bay leaves
- Salt and ground black pepper, to taste
- 3 tablespoons fresh parsley, chopped
- 1 onion, peeled and chopped
- 1 teaspoon dried sage
- 1 tablespoon garlic, minced
- 2 cups water

Directions:
Heat up a pan with 1 teaspoon oil over medium heat, add the beef, stir, and brown for 10 minutes. In a pot, mix the chicken, beef stock, sauerkraut, stevia, canned tomatoes, Worcestershire sauce, parsley, sage, and bay leaves, stir, and bring to a simmer over medium heat. Add the beef to soup, stir, and continue simmering. Heat up the same pan with the rest of the oil over medium heat, add the onions, stir, and cook for 2 minutes. Add the garlic, stir, cook for 1 minute, and add this to the soup. Reduce heat to soup, and simmer it for 1 hour. Add the salt, pepper, and water, stir, and cook for 15 minutes. Divide into bowls and serve.

Nutrition: Calories - 250, Fat - 5, Fiber - 1, Carbs - 3, Protein - 12

Ground Beef Casserole

Preparation time: 10 minutes
Cooking time: 35 minutes
Servings: 6

Ingredients:
- 2 teaspoons onion flakes
- 1 tablespoon gluten-free Worcestershire sauce
- 2 pounds ground beef
- 2 garlic cloves, peeled and minced
- Salt and ground black pepper, to taste
- 1 cup mozzarella cheese, shredded
- 2 cups cheddar cheese, shredded
- 1 cup Russian dressing
- 2 tablespoons sesame seeds, toasted
- 20 dill pickle slices
- 1 romaine lettuce head, torn

Directions:
Heat up a pan over medium heat, add the beef, onion flakes, Worcestershire sauce, salt, pepper, and garlic, stir, and cook for 5 minutes. Transfer this to a baking dish, add the 1 cup cheddar cheese, mozzarella cheese, and half of the Russian dressing. Stir and spread evenly. Arrange the pickle slices on top, sprinkle the rest of the cheddar and the sesame seeds, place in an oven at 350ºF, and bake for 20 minutes. Turn the oven to broil and broil the casserole for 5 minutes. Divide lettuce on plates, top with a beef casserole, and the rest of the Russian dressing.

Nutrition: Calories - 554, Fat - 51, Fiber - 3, Carbs - 5, Protein - 45

Zucchini Noodles and Beef

Preparation time: 10 minutes
Cooking time: 20 minutes
Servings: 5

Ingredients:
- 1 pound ground beef
- 1 onion, peeled and chopped
- 2 garlic cloves, peeled and minced
- 14 ounces canned diced tomatoes
- 1 tablespoon dried rosemary
- 1 tablespoon dried sage
- 1 tablespoon dried oregano
- 1 tablespoon dried basil
- 1 tablespoon dried marjoram
- Salt and ground black pepper, to taste
- 2 zucchini, cut with a spiralizer

Directions:
Heat up a pan over medium heat, add the garlic and onion, stir, and brown for a couple of minutes. Add the beef, stir, and cook for 6 minutes. Add the tomatoes, salt, pepper, rosemary, sage, oregano, marjoram, and basil, stir, and simmer for 15 minutes. Divide the zucchini noodles into bowls, add the beef mixture, and serve.

Nutrition: Calories - 320, Fat - 13, Fiber - 4, Carbs - 12, Protein - 40

Jamaican Beef Pies

Preparation time: 10 minutes
Cooking time: 35 minutes
Servings: 12

Ingredients:
- 3 garlic cloves, peeled and minced
- ½ pound ground beef
- ½ pound ground pork
- ½ cup water
- 1 small onion, peeled and chopped
- 2 habanero peppers, chopped
- 1 teaspoon Jamaican curry powder
- 1 teaspoon dried thyme
- 2 teaspoons coriander
- ½ teaspoon allspice
- 2 teaspoons cumin
- ½ teaspoon turmeric
- A pinch of ground cloves
- Salt and ground black pepper, to taste
- 1 teaspoon garlic powder
- ¼ teaspoon stevia powder
- 2 tablespoons butter

For the crust:
- 4 tablespoons butter, melted
- 6 ounces cream cheese
- A pinch of salt
- 1 teaspoon turmeric
- ¼ teaspoon stevia
- ½ teaspoon baking powder
- 1½ cups flax meal
- 2 tablespoons water
- ½ cup coconut flour

Directions:
In a blender, mix onion with habaneros, garlic, and ½ cup water. Heat up a pan over medium heat, add the pork and beef, stir, and cook for 3 minutes. Add the onions mixture, stir, and cook for 2 minutes. Add the garlic, onion, curry powder, ½ teaspoon turmeric, thyme, coriander, cumin, allspice, cloves, salt, pepper, stevia powder, and garlic powder, stir well, and cook for 3 minutes. Add the 2 tablespoons butter, stir until it melts, and take this off heat. In a bowl, mix the 1 teaspoon turmeric, with ¼ teaspoon stevia, baking powder, flax meal, and coconut flour, and stir. In a separate bowl, mix the 4 tablespoons butter with 2 tablespoons water, and cream cheese, and stir. Combine the 2 mixtures, and mix until you obtain a dough. Shape 12 balls from this mixture, place them on a parchment paper, and roll each into a circle. Divide the beef and pork mix on one half of the dough circles, cover with the other half, seal edges, and arrange them all on a lined baking sheet. Bake the pies in the oven at 350°F for 25 minutes. Serve warm.

Nutrition: Calories - 267, Fat - 23, Fiber - 1, Carbs - 3, Protein - 12

Beef Goulash

Preparation time: 10 minutes
Cooking time: 20 minutes
Servings: 5

Ingredients:
- 2 ounces bell pepper, seeded and chopped
- 1½ pounds ground beef
- Salt and ground black pepper, to taste
- 2 cups cauliflower florets
- ¼ cup onion, peeled and chopped
- 14 ounces canned diced tomatoes, and
- ¼ teaspoon garlic powder
- 1 tablespoon tomato paste
- 14 ounces water

Directions:
Heat up a pan over medium heat, add the beef, stir, and brown for 5 minutes. Add the onion and bell pepper, stir, and cook for 4 minutes. Add the cauliflower, tomatoes, and water, stir, bring to a simmer, cover pan, and cook for 5 minutes. Add the tomato paste, garlic powder, salt, and pepper, stir, take off the heat, divide into bowls, and serve.

Nutrition: Calories - 275, Fat - 7, Fiber - 2, Carbs - 4, Protein - 10

Beef and Eggplant Casserole

Preparation time: 30 minutes
Cooking time: 4 hours
Servings: 12

Ingredients:
- 1 tablespoon olive oil
- 2 pounds ground beef
- 2 cups eggplant, chopped
- Salt and ground black pepper, to taste
- 2 teaspoons mustard
- 2 teaspoons gluten-free Worcestershire sauce
- 28 ounces canned diced tomatoes
- 2 cups mozzarella cheese, grated
- 16 ounces tomato sauce
- 2 tablespoons fresh parsley, chopped
- 1 teaspoon dried oregano

Directions:
Season the eggplant pieces with salt and pepper, set them aside for 30 minutes, squeeze water a bit, put them into a bowl, add the olive oil, and toss them to coat. In another bowl, mix the beef with salt, pepper, mustard, and Worcestershire sauce, and stir well. Press them on the bottom of a slow cooker. Add the eggplant and spread the pieces out. Add the tomatoes, tomato sauce, parsley, oregano, and mozzarella cheese. Cover the slow cooker, and cook on low for 4 hours. Divide the casserole on plates and serve hot.

Nutrition: Calories - 200, Fat - 12, Fiber - 2, Carbs - 6, Protein - 15

Braised Lamb Chops

Preparation time: 10 minutes
Cooking time: 2 hours and 20 minutes
Servings: 4

Ingredients:
- 8 lamb chops
- 1 teaspoon garlic powder
- Salt and ground black pepper, to taste
- 2 teaspoons fresh mint, crushed
- A drizzle of olive oil
- 1 shallot, peeled and chopped
- 1 cup white wine
- Juice of ½ lemon
- 1 bay leaf
- 2 cups beef stock
- Fresh parsley, chopped, for serving

For the sauce:
- 2 cups cranberries
- ½ teaspoon fresh rosemary, chopped
- ½ cup swerve
- 1 teaspoon dried mint
- Juice of ½ lemon
- 1 teaspoon fresh ginger, grated
- 1 cup water
- 1 teaspoon harissa paste

Directions:
In a bowl, mix the lamb chops with salt, pepper, 1 teaspoon garlic powder, and 2 teaspoons mint, and rub well. Heat up a pan with a drizzle of oil over medium-high heat, add the lamb chops, brown them on all sides, and transfer to a plate. Heat up the same pan again over medium-high heat, add the shallots, stir, and cook for 1 minute. Add the wine and bay leaf, stir, and cook for 4 minutes. Add the 2 cups beef stock, parsley, and juice from ½ lemon, stir, and simmer for 5 minutes. Return the lamb, stir, and cook for 10 minutes. Cover the pan, and place it in the oven at 350ºF for 2 hours. Heat up a pan over medium-high heat, add the cranberries, swerve, rosemary, 1 teaspoon mint, juice from ½ lemon, ginger, water, and harissa paste, stir, bring to a simmer for 15 minutes. Take the lamb chops out of the oven, divide them on plates, drizzle the cranberry sauce over them, and serve.

Nutrition: Calories - 450, Fat - 34, Fiber - 2, Carbs - 6, Protein - 26

Lamb Salad

Preparation time: 10 minutes
Cooking time: 35 minutes
Servings: 4

Ingredients:
- 1 tablespoon olive oil
- 3 pounds leg of lamb, bone removed, and leg butterflied
- Salt and ground black pepper, to taste
- 1 teaspoon cumin
- A pinch of dried thyme
- 2 garlic cloves, peeled and minced

For the salad:
- 4 ounces feta cheese, crumbled
- ½ cup pecans
- 2 cups spinach
- 1½ tablespoons lemon juice
- ¼ cup olive oil
- 1 cup fresh mint, chopped

Directions:
Rub the lamb with salt, pepper, 1 tablespoon oil, thyme, cumin, and minced garlic, place on preheated grill over medium-high heat, and cook for 40 minutes, flipping once. Spread the pecans on a lined baking sheet, place in an oven at 350ºF, and toast for 10 minutes. Transfer the grilled lamb to a cutting board, set aside to cool down, and slice. In a salad bowl, mix the spinach with 1 cup mint, feta cheese, ¼ cup olive oil, lemon juice, toasted pecans, salt, and pepper, and toss to coat. Add the lamb slices on top and serve.

Nutrition: Calories - 334, Fat - 33, Fiber - 3, Carbs - 5, Protein - 7

Moroccan Lamb

Preparation time: 10 minutes
Cooking time: 15 minutes
Servings: 4

Ingredients:

- 2 teaspoons paprika
- 2 garlic cloves, peeled and minced
- 2 teaspoons dried oregano
- 2 tablespoons sumac
- 12 lamb cutlets
- ¼ cup olive oil
- 2 tablespoons water
- 2 teaspoons cumin
- 4 carrots, peeled, and sliced
- ¼ cup fresh parsley, chopped
- 2 teaspoons harissa
- 1 tablespoon red wine vinegar
- Salt and ground black pepper, to taste
- 2 tablespoons black olives, pitted and sliced
- 6 radishes, sliced thin

Directions:

In a bowl, mix the cutlets with the paprika, garlic, oregano, sumac, salt, pepper, half of the oil, and the water, and rub well. Put the carrots in a pot, add the water to cover, bring to a boil over medium-high heat, cook for 2 minutes drain, and put them in a salad bowl. Add the olives and radishes to the carrots. In another bowl, mix the harissa with the rest of the oil, parsley, cumin, vinegar, and a splash of water, and stir well. Add this to the carrots mixture, season with salt and pepper, and toss to coat. Heat up a kitchen grill over medium-high heat, add the lamb cutlets, grill them for 3 minutes on each side, and divide them on plates. Add the carrot salad on the side and serve.

Nutrition: Calories - 245, Fat - 32, Fiber - 6, Carbs - 4, Protein - 34

Lamb with Mustard Sauce

Preparation time: 10 minutes
Cooking time: 20 minutes
Servings: 4

Ingredients:

- 2 tablespoons olive oil
- 1 tablespoon fresh rosemary, chopped
- 2 garlic cloves, peeled and minced
- 1½ pounds lamb chops
- Salt and ground black pepper, to taste
- 1 tablespoon shallot, peeled and chopped
- ⅔ cup heavy cream
- ½ cup beef stock
- 1 tablespoon mustard
- 2 teaspoons gluten-free Worcestershire sauce
- 2 teaspoons lemon juice
- 1 teaspoon erythritol
- 2 tablespoons butter
- A sprig of rosemary
- A sprig of thyme

Directions:

In a bowl, mix the 1 tablespoon oil with the garlic, salt, pepper, and rosemary, and whisk. Add the lamb chops, toss to coat, and set aside for a few minutes. Heat up a pan with the rest of the oil over medium-high heat, add the lamb chops, reduce heat to medium, cook them for 7 minutes, flip, cook them for 7 minutes, transfer to a plate, and keep them warm. Return the pan to medium heat, add the shallots, stir, and cook for 3 minutes. Add the stock, stir, and cook for 1 minute. Add the Worcestershire sauce, mustard, erythritol, cream, rosemary, and thyme, stir, and cook for 8 minutes. Add the lemon juice, salt, pepper, and the butter, discard the rosemary and thyme, stir well, and take off the heat. Divide the lamb chops on plates, drizzle the sauce over them, and serve.

Nutrition: Calories - 435, Fat - 30, Fiber - 4, Carbs - 5, Protein - 32

Lamb Curry

Preparation time: 10 minutes
Cooking time: 4 hours
Servings: 6

Ingredients:
- 2 tablespoons fresh ginger, grated
- 2 garlic cloves, peeled and minced
- 2 teaspoons cardamom
- 1 onion, peeled and chopped
- 6 cloves
- 1 pound lamb meat, cubed
- 2 teaspoons cumin powder
- 1 teaspoon garam masala
- ½ teaspoon chili powder
- 1 teaspoon turmeric
- 2 teaspoons coriander
- 1 pound spinach
- 14 ounces canned diced tomatoes

Directions:
In a slow cooker, mix the lamb with the spinach, tomatoes, ginger, garlic, onion, cardamom, cloves, cumin, garam masala, chili, turmeric, and coriander, stir, cover, and cook on high for 4 hours. Uncover the slow cooker, stir the chili, divide into bowls, and serve.

Nutrition: Calories - 160, Fat - 6, Fiber - 3, Carbs - 7, Protein - 20

Lamb Stew

Preparation time: 10 minutes
Cooking time: 3 hours
Servings: 4

Ingredients:
- 1 onion, peeled and chopped
- 3 carrots, peeled and chopped
- 2 pounds lamb, cubed
- 1 tomato, cored and chopped
- 1 garlic clove, peeled and minced
- 2 tablespoons butter
- 1 cup beef stock
- 1 cup white wine
- Salt and ground black pepper, to taste
- 2 rosemary sprigs
- 1 teaspoon fresh thyme, chopped

Directions:
Heat up a Dutch oven over medium-high heat, add the oil, and heat up. Add the lamb, salt, and pepper, brown on all sides, and transfer to a plate. Add the onion to the Dutch oven and cook for 2 minutes. Add the carrots, tomato, garlic, butter, stick, wine, salt, pepper, rosemary, and thyme, stir, and cook for a couple of minutes. Return the lamb to Dutch oven, stir, reduce heat to medium-low, cover, and cook for 4 hours. Discard the rosemary sprigs, add more salt and pepper, stir, divide into bowls, and serve.

Nutrition: Calories - 700, Fat - 43, Fiber - 6, Carbs - 10, Protein - 67

Lamb Casserole

Preparation time: 10 minutes
Cooking time: 1 hour and 40 minutes
Servings: 2

Ingredients:
- 2 garlic cloves, peeled and minced
- 1 onion, peeled and chopped
- 1 tablespoon olive oil
- 1 celery stalk, chopped
- 10 ounces lamb fillet, cut into medium-sized pieces
- Salt and ground black pepper, to taste
- 1¼ cups lamb stock
- 2 carrots, peeled and chopped
- ½ tablespoon fresh rosemary, chopped
- 1 leek, chopped
- 1 tablespoon mint sauce
- 1 teaspoon stevia
- 1 tablespoon tomato puree
- ½ cauliflower, separated into florets
- ½ celeriac, chopped
- 2 tablespoons butter

Directions:
Heat up a pot with the oil over medium heat, add the garlic, onion, and celery, stir, and cook for 5 minutes. Add the lamb pieces, stir, and cook for 3 minutes. Add the carrot, leek, rosemary, stock, tomato puree, mint sauce, and stevia, stir, bring to a boil, cover, and cook for 1 hour and 30 minutes. Heat up a pot with water over medium heat, add the celeriac, cover, and simmer for 10 minutes. Add the cauliflower florets, cook for 15 minutes, drain everything, and mix with salt, pepper, and butter. Mash using a potato masher, and divide the mash on plates. Add the lamb and vegetables mixture on top and serve.

Nutrition: Calories - 324, Fat - 4, Fiber - 5, Carbs - 8, Protein - 20

Slow-cooked Leg of Lamb

Preparation time: 10 minutes
Cooking time: 8 hours
Servings: 6

Ingredients:
- 2 pounds lamb leg
- Salt and ground black pepper, to taste
- 1 tablespoon maple extract
- 2 tablespoons mustard
- ¼ cup olive oil
- 4 thyme sprigs
- 6 mint leaves
- 1 teaspoon garlic, minced
- A pinch of dried rosemary

Directions:
Put the oil in a slow cooker. Add the lamb, salt, pepper, maple extract, mustard, rosemary, and garlic, rub well, cover, and cook on low for 7 hours. Add the mint and thyme, and cook for 1 hour. Let the lamb to cool before slicing and serving with pan juices on top.

Nutrition: Calories - 400, Fat - 34, Fiber - 1, Carbs - 3, Protein - 26

Lavender Lamb Chops

Preparation time: 10 minutes
Cooking time: 25 minutes
Servings: 4

Ingredients:
- 2 tablespoons rosemary, chopped
- 1½ pounds lamb chops
- Salt and ground black pepper, to taste
- 1 tablespoon fresh lavender, chopped
- 2 garlic cloves, peeled and minced
- 3 red oranges, cut in half
- 2 small pieces of orange peel
- A drizzle of olive oil
- 1 teaspoon butter

Directions:
In a bowl, mix the lamb chops with salt, pepper, rosemary, lavender, garlic, and orange peel, toss to coat, and set aside for a couple of hours. Grease a kitchen grill with butter, heat up over medium-high heat, place lamb chops on it, cook for 3 minutes, flip, squeeze 1 orange half over them, cook for 3 minutes, flip them again, cook them for 2 minutes, and squeeze another orange half over them. Place the lamb chops on a plate and keep them warm for now. Add the remaining orange half on preheated grill, cook them for 3 minutes, flip, and cook them for another 3 minutes. Divide the lamb chops on plates, add the orange half on the side, drizzle some olive oil over them, and serve.

Nutrition: Calories - 250, Fat - 5, Fiber - 1, Carbs - 5, Protein – 8

Paprika Lamb Chops

Preparation time: 10 minutes
Cooking time: 15 minutes
Servings: 4

Ingredients:
- 2 lamb racks, cut into chops
- Salt and ground black pepper, to taste
- 3 tablespoons paprika
- ¾ cup cumin powder
- 1 teaspoon chili powder

Directions:
In a bowl, mix the paprika with cumin, chili, salt, and pepper, and stir. Add the lamb chops and rub them well. Heat up a grill over medium temperature, add the lamb chops, cook for 5 minutes, flip, and cook for 5 minutes. Flip them again, cook for 2 minutes, and then for 2 minutes on the other side again.

Nutrition: Calories - 200, Fat - 5, Fiber - 2, Carbs - 4, Protein - 8

Lamb with Orange Dressing

Preparation time: 10 minutes
Cooking time: 4 hours
Servings: 4

Ingredients:
- 2 lamb shanks
- Salt and ground black pepper, to taste
- 1 garlic head, peeled
- 4 tablespoons olive oil
- Juice of ½ lemon
- Zest from ½ lemon
- ½ teaspoon dried oregano

Directions:
In a slow cooker, mix the lamb with salt and pepper. Add the garlic, cover, and cook on high for 4 hours.
In a bowl, mix the lemon juice with lemon zest, some salt and pepper, the olive oil, and oregano, and whisk. Uncover the slow cooker, shred the lamb, discard the bone, and divide on plates. Drizzle the lemon dressing all over and serve.

Nutrition: Calories - 160, Fat - 7, Fiber - 3, Carbs - 5, Protein - 12

Lamb Riblets and Mint Pesto

Preparation time: 1 hour
Cooking time: 2 hours
Servings: 4

Ingredients:
- 1 cup parsley
- 1 cup mint
- 1½ onions, peeled and chopped
- ⅓ cup pistachios
- 1 teaspoon lemon zest
- 5 tablespoons avocado oil
- Salt, to taste
- 2 pounds lamb riblets
- 5 garlic cloves, peeled and minced
- Juice from 1 orange

Directions:
In a food processor, mix the parsley with mint, 1 onion, pistachios, lemon zest, salt, and avocado oil, and blend well. Rub the lamb with this mixture, place in a bowl, cover, and leave in the refrigerator for 1 hour. Transfer the lamb to a baking dish, add the garlic, and ½ onion to the dish as well, drizzle with orange juice, and bake in the oven at 250°F for 2 hours. Divide on plates and serve.

Nutrition: Calories - 200, Fat - 4, Fiber - 1, Carbs - 5, Protein - 7

Lamb with Fennel and Figs

Preparation time: 10 minutes
Cooking time: 40 minutes
Servings: 4

Ingredients:
- 12 ounces lamb racks
- 2 fennel bulbs, sliced
- Salt and ground black pepper, to taste
- 2 tablespoons olive oil
- 4 figs, cut in half
- ⅛ cup apple cider vinegar
- 1 tablespoon swerve

Directions:
In a bowl, mix the fennel with figs, vinegar, swerve, and oil, toss to coat well, and transfer to a baking dish. Season with salt and pepper, place in an oven at 400°F, and bake for 15 minutes. Season the lamb with salt and pepper, place into a heated pan over medium-high heat, and cook for a couple of minutes. Add the lamb to the baking dish with the fennel and figs, place in an oven, and bake for 20 minutes. Divide everything on plates and serve.

Nutrition: Calories - 230, Fat - 3, Fiber - 3, Carbs - 5, Protein - 10

Baked Veal and Cabbage

Preparation time: 10 minutes
Cooking time: 40 minutes
Servings: 4

Ingredients:
- 17 ounces veal, cut into cubes
- 1 cabbage head, shredded
- Salt and ground black pepper, to taste
- 3. 4 ounces ham, chopped
- 1 onion, peeled and chopped
- 2 garlic cloves, peeled and minced
- 1 tablespoon butter
- ½ cup Parmesan cheese, grated
- ½ cup sour cream

Directions:
Heat up a pot with the butter over medium-high heat, add the onion, stir, and cook for 2 minutes. Add the garlic, stir, and cook for 1 minute. Add the ham and veal, stir and cook until slightly browned. Add the cabbage, stir and cook until it softens, and the meat is tender. Add the cream, salt, pepper, and cheese, stir gently, place in an oven at 350°F, and bake for 20 minutes. Divide on plates and serve.

Nutrition: Calories - 230, Fat - 7, Fiber - 4, Carbs - 6, Protein - 29

Beef Bourguignon

Preparation time: 3 hours and 10 minutes
Cooking time: 5 hours and 15 minutes
Servings: 8

Ingredients:
- 3 tablespoons olive oil
- 2 tablespoons onion, peeled and chopped
- 1 tablespoon dried parsley flakes
- 1½ cups red wine
- 1 teaspoon dried thyme
- Salt and ground black pepper, to taste
- 1 bay leaf
- ⅓ cup almond flour
- 4 pounds beef, cubed
- 24 small white onions
- 8 bacon slices, chopped
- 2 garlic cloves, peeled and minced
- 1 pound mushrooms, chopped

Directions:
In a bowl, mix the wine with olive oil, minced onion, thyme, parsley, salt, pepper, and bay leaf, and whisk. Add the beef cubes, stir, and set aside for 3 hours. Drain the meat, and reserve 1 cup of marinade. Add the flour over meat, and toss to coat. Heat up a pan over medium-high heat, add the bacon, stir and cook slightly browned. Add the onions, stir, and cook for 3 minutes. Add the garlic, stir, cook for 1 minute, and transfer everything to a slow cooker. Add the meat to the slow cooker and stir. Heat up the pan with the bacon fat over medium-high heat, add the mushrooms and onions, stir, and sauté them for a couple of minutes. Add these to the slow cooker as well with the reserved marinade, some salt and pepper, cover, and cook on high for 5 hours. Divide on plates and serve.

Nutrition: Calories - 435, Fat - 16, Fiber - 1, Carbs - 7, Protein - 45

Slow-roasted Beef

Preparation time: 10 minutes
Cooking time: 8 hours
Servings: 8

Ingredients:
- 5 pounds beef roast
- Salt and ground black pepper, to taste
- ½ teaspoon celery salt
- 2 teaspoons chili powder
- 1 tablespoon avocado oil
- 1 tablespoon sweet paprika
- A pinch of cayenne pepper
- ½ teaspoon garlic powder
- ½ cup beef stock
- 1 tablespoon garlic, minced
- ¼ teaspoon dry mustard

Directions:
Heat up a pan with the oil over medium-high heat, add the beef roast, and brown it on all sides. In a bowl, mix the paprika with chili powder, celery salt, salt, pepper, cayenne, garlic powder, and dry mustard, and stir. Add the roast, rub well, and transfer it to a slow cooker. Add the beef stock and garlic over roast, and cook on low for 8 hours. Transfer the beef to a cutting board, leave it to cool, slice, and divide on plates. Strain the juices from the pot, drizzle over the meat, and serve.

Nutrition: Calories - 180, Fat - 5, Fiber - 1, Carbs - 5, Protein - 25

Beef Stew

Preparation time: 10 minutes
Cooking time: 4 hours and 10 minutes
Servings: 4

Ingredients:
- 8 ounces pancetta, chopped
- 4 pounds beef, cubed
- 4 garlic cloves, peeled and minced
- 2 brown onions, peeled and chopped
- 2 tablespoons olive oil
- 4 tablespoons red vinegar
- 4 cups beef stock
- 2 tablespoons tomato paste
- 2 cinnamon sticks
- 3 lemon peel strips
- ½ cup fresh parsley, chopped
- 4 thyme sprigs
- 2 tablespoons butter
- Salt and ground black pepper, to taste

Directions:
Heat up a pan with the oil over medium-high heat, add the pancetta, onion, and garlic, stir, and cook for 5 minutes. Add the beef, stir, and cook until it browns. Add the vinegar, salt, pepper, stock, tomato paste, cinnamon, lemon peel, thyme, and butter, stir, cook for 3 minutes, and transfer everything to a slow cooker. Cover and cook on high for 4 hours. Discard the cinnamon, lemon peel, and thyme, add the parsley, stir, and divide into bowls. Serve hot.

Nutrition: Calories - 250, Fat - 6, Fiber - 1, Carbs - 7, Protein - 33

Pork Stew

Preparation time: 10 minutes
Cooking time: 1 hour and 20 minutes
Servings: 12

Ingredients:
- 2 tablespoons coconut oil
- 4 pounds pork, cubed
- Salt and ground black pepper, to taste
- 2 tablespoons butter
- 3 garlic cloves, peeled and minced
- ¾ cup beef stock
- ¾ cup apple cider vinegar
- 3 carrots, peeled and chopped
- 1 cabbage head, shredded
- ½ cup green onion, chopped
- 1 cup heavy cream

Directions:
Heat up a pan with the butter and oil over medium-high heat, add the pork and brown it for a few minutes on each side. Add the vinegar and stock, stir well, and bring to a simmer. Add the cabbage, garlic, salt, and pepper, stir, cover, and cook for 1 hour. Add the carrots and green onions, stir, and cook for 15 minutes. Add the heavy cream, stir for 1 minute, divide on plates, and serve.

Nutrition: Calories - 400, Fat - 25, Fiber - 3, Carbs - 6, Protein - 43

Sausage Stew

Preparation time: 10 minutes
Cooking time: 20 minutes
Servings: 9

Ingredients:
- 1 pound smoked sausage, sliced
- 1 green bell pepper, seeded and chopped
- 2 onions, peeled and chopped
- Salt and ground black pepper, to taste
- 1 cup fresh parsley, chopped
- 8 green onions, chopped
- ¼ cup avocado oil
- 1 cup beef stock
- 6 garlic cloves
- 28 ounces canned diced tomatoes
- 16 ounces okra, trimmed and sliced
- 8 ounces tomato sauce
- 2 tablespoons coconut aminos
- 1 tablespoon gluten-free hot sauce

Directions:
Heat up a pot with the oil over medium-high heat, add the sausages, stir, and cook for 2 minutes. Add the onion, bell pepper, green onions, parsley, salt, and pepper, stir, and cook for 2 minutes. Add the stock, garlic, tomatoes, okra, tomato sauce, coconut aminos, and hot sauce, stir, bring to a simmer, and cook for 15 minutes. Add more salt, and pepper, stir, divide into bowls, and serve.

Nutrition: Calories - 274, Fat - 20, Fiber - 4, Carbs - 7, Protein - 10

Burgundy Beef Stew

Preparation time: 10 minutes
Cooking time: 3 hours
Servings: 7

Ingredients:
- 2 pounds beef chuck roast, cubed
- 15 ounces canned diced tomatoes
- 4 carrots, peeled and chopped
- Salt and ground black pepper, to taste
- ½ pounds mushrooms, sliced
- 2 celery stalks, chopped
- 2 onions, peeled and chopped
- 1 cup beef stock
- 1 tablespoon fresh thyme, chopped
- ½ teaspoon dry mustard
- 3 tablespoons almond flour
- 1 cup water

Directions:
Heat up an ovenproof pot over medium-high heat, add the beef cubes, stir, and brown them for a couple of minutes on each side. Add the tomatoes, mushrooms, onions, carrots, celery, salt, pepper mustard, stock, and thyme, and stir. In a bowl, mix the water with flour and stir well. Add this to the pot, stir well, place in an oven, and bake at 325°F for 3 hours. Stir every 30 minutes. Divide into bowls and serve.

Nutrition: Calories - 275, Fat - 13, Fiber - 4, Carbs - 7, Protein - 28

Cuban Beef Stew

Preparation time: 10 minutes
Cooking time: 6 hours
Servings: 8

Ingredients:
- 2 onions, peeled and chopped
- 2 tablespoons avocado oil
- 2 pounds beef roast, cubed
- 2 green bell peppers, seeded and chopped
- 1 habanero pepper, chopped
- 4 jalapeños, chopped
- 14 ounces canned diced tomatoes
- 2 tablespoons fresh cilantro, chopped
- 6 garlic cloves, peeled and minced
- ½ cup water
- Salt and ground black pepper, to taste
- 1½ teaspoons cumin
- 4 teaspoons bouillon granules
- ½ cup black olives, pitted and chopped
- 1 teaspoon dried oregano

Directions:
Heat up a pan with the oil over medium-high heat, add the beef, brown it on all sides, and transfer to a slow cooker. Add the green bell peppers, onions, jalapeños, habanero pepper, tomatoes, garlic, water, bouillon, cilantro, oregano, cumin, salt, and pepper, and stir. Cover the slow cooker, and cook on low for 6 hours. Add the olives, stir, divide into bowls, and serve.

Nutrition: Calories - 305, Fat - 14, Fiber - 4, Carbs - 8, Protein - 25

Ham Stew

Preparation time: 10 minutes
Cooking time: 4 hours
Servings: 6

Ingredients:
- 8 ounces cheddar cheese, grated
- 14 ounces chicken stock
- ½ teaspoon garlic powder
- ½ teaspoon onion powder
- Salt and ground black pepper, to taste
- 4 garlic cloves, peeled and minced
- ¼ cup heavy cream
- 3 cups ham, chopped
- 16 ounces cauliflower florets

Directions:
In a slow cooker, mix the ham with stock, cheese, cauliflower, garlic powder, onion powder, salt, pepper, garlic, and heavy cream, stir, cover, and cook on high for 4 hours. Stir, divide into bowls, and serve.

Nutrition: Calories - 320, Fat - 20, Fiber - 3, Carbs - 6, Protein - 23

Veal Stew

Preparation time: 10 minutes
Cooking time: 2 hours and 10 minutes
Servings: 12

Ingredients:
- 2 tablespoons avocado oil
- 3 pounds veal, cubed
- 1 onion, peeled and chopped
- 1 garlic clove, peeled and minced
- Salt and ground black pepper, to taste
- 1 cup water
- 1½ cups marsala wine
- 10 ounces canned tomato paste
- 1 carrot, peeled, and chopped
- 7 ounces mushrooms, chopped
- 3 egg yolks
- ½ cup heavy cream
- 2 teaspoons dried oregano

Directions:
Heat up a pot with the oil over medium-high heat, add the veal, stir, and brown it for a few minutes. Add the garlic and onion, stir, and cook for 2-3 minutes. Add the wine, water, oregano, tomato paste, mushrooms, carrots, salt, and pepper, stir, bring to a boil, cover, reduce the heat to low, and cook for 1 hour and 45 minutes. In a bowl, mix the cream with egg yolks, and whisk. Pour this into the pot, stir, cook for 15 minutes, add more salt and pepper, if needed, divide into bowls, and serve.

Nutrition: Calories - 254, Fat - 15, Fiber - 1, Carbs - 3, Protein - 23

Veal with Tomatoes

Preparation time: 10 minutes
Cooking time: 40 minutes
Servings: 4

Ingredients:
- 4 medium veal leg steaks
- A drizzle of avocado oil
- 2 garlic cloves, peeled and minced
- 1 onion, peeled and chopped
- Salt and ground black pepper, to taste
- 2 teaspoons fresh sage, chopped
- 15 ounces canned diced tomatoes
- 2 tablespoons fresh parsley, chopped
- 1 ounce semi-soft cheese, sliced
- Green beans, steamed, for serving

Directions:
Heat up a pan with the oil over medium-high heat, add the veal, cook for 2 minutes on each side, and transfer to a baking dish. Return the pan to heat, add the onion, stir, and cook for 4 minutes. Add the sage and garlic, stir, and cook for 1 minute. Add the tomatoes, stir, bring to a boil, and cook for 10 minutes. Pour this over the veal, add the cheese and parsley, place in an oven at 350°F, and bake for 20 minutes. Divide on plates and serve.

Nutrition: Calories - 276, Fat - 6, Fiber - 4, Carbs - 5, Protein - 36

Veal Parmesan

Preparation time: 10 minutes
Cooking time: 1 hour and 10 minutes
Servings: 6

Ingredients:
- 8 veal cutlets
- ⅔ cup Parmesan cheese, grated
- 8 provolone cheese slices
- Salt and ground black pepper, to taste
- 5 cups tomato sauce
- A pinch of garlic salt
- Vegetable oil cooking spray
- 2 tablespoons butter
- 2 tablespoons coconut oil, melted
- 1 teaspoon Italian seasoning

Directions:
Season the veal cutlets with salt, pepper, and garlic salt. Heat up a pan with the butter and oil over medium-high heat, add the veal, and cook until they brown on all sides. Spread half of the tomato sauce on the bottom of a baking dish which you've coated with some cooking spray. Add the veal cutlets, then sprinkle with Italian seasoning and spread the rest of the sauce. Cover the dish, place in an oven at 350°F, and bake for 40 minutes. Uncover the dish, spread with the provolone cheese, sprinkle with the Parmesan cheese, place in an oven again, and bake for 15 minutes. Divide on plates and serve.

Nutrition: Calories - 362, Fat - 21, Fiber - 2, Carbs - 6, Protein - 26

Veal Piccata

Preparation time: 10 minutes
Cooking time: 15 minutes
Servings: 2

Ingredients:
- 2 tablespoons butter
- ¼ cup white wine
- ¼ cup chicken stock
- 1½ tablespoons capers
- 1 garlic clove, peeled and minced
- 8 ounces veal scallops
- Salt and ground black pepper, to taste

Directions:
Heat up a pan with half of the butter over medium-high heat, add the veal cutlets, season with salt and pepper, cook for 1 minute on each side, and transfer to a plate. Heat up the pan again over medium heat, add the garlic, stir, and cook for 1 minute. Add the wine, stir, and simmer for 2 minutes. Add the stock, capers, salt, pepper, the rest of the butter, and return the veal to pan. Stir everything, cover the pan, and cook piccata on medium-low heat until veal is tender.

Nutrition: Calories - 204, Fat - 12, Fiber - 1, Carbs - 5, Protein - 10

Roasted Pork Sausage

Preparation time: 10 minutes
Cooking time: 1 hour
Servings: 6

Ingredients:
- 3 red bell peppers, seeded and chopped
- 2 pounds Italian pork sausage, sliced
- Salt and ground black pepper, to taste
- 2 pounds Portobello mushrooms, sliced
- 2 sweet onions, peeled and chopped
- 1 tablespoon swerve
- A drizzle of olive oil

Directions:
In a baking dish, mix the sausage slices with oil, salt, pepper, bell pepper, mushrooms, onion, and swerve. Toss to coat, place in an oven at 300ºF, and bake for 1 hour. Divide on plates and serve hot.

Nutrition: Calories - 130, Fat - 12, Fiber - 1, Carbs - 3, Protein - 9

Baked Sausage and Kale

Preparation time: 5 minutes
Cooking time: 30 minutes
Servings: 4

Ingredients:
- 1 cup onion, peeled and chopped
- 1½ pound Italian pork sausage, sliced
- ½ cup red bell pepper, seeded and chopped
- Salt and ground black pepper, to taste
- 5 pounds kale, chopped
- 1 teaspoon garlic, minced
- ¼ cup red chili pepper, chopped
- 1 cup water

Directions:
Heat up a pan over medium-high heat, add the sausage, stir, reduce heat to medium, and cook for 10 minutes.
Add the onions, stir, and cook for 3-4 minutes. Add the bell pepper and garlic, stir, and cook for 1 minute. Add the kale, chili pepper, salt, pepper, and water, stir, and cook for 10 minutes. Divide on plates and serve.

Nutrition: Calories - 150, Fat - 4, Fiber - 1, Carbs - 2, Protein - 12

Sausage with Tomatoes and Cheese

Preparation time: 10 minutes
Cooking time: 30 minutes
Servings: 4

Ingredients:
- 2 ounces coconut oil, melted
- 2 pounds Italian pork sausage, chopped
- 1 onion, peeled and sliced
- 4 sundried tomatoes, sliced thin
- Salt and ground black pepper, to taste
- ½ pound gouda cheese, grated
- 3 yellow bell peppers, seeded and chopped
- 3 orange bell peppers, seeded and chopped
- A pinch of red pepper flakes
- ½ cup parsley, sliced thin

Directions:
Heat up a pan with the oil over medium-high heat, add the sausage slices, stir, cook for 3 minutes on each side, transfer to a plate, and set aside. Heat up the pan again over medium heat, add the onion, bell peppers, and tomatoes, stir, and cook for 5 minutes. Add the pepper flakes, salt, and pepper, stir well, cook for 1 minute, and take off the heat. Arrange the sausage slices into a baking dish, add the bell peppers mixture on top, add the parsley and Gouda cheese, place in an oven at 350ºF, and bake for 15 minutes. Divide on plates and serve hot.

Nutrition: Calories - 200, Fat - 5, Fiber - 3, Carbs - 6, Protein - 14

Sausage Salad

Preparation time: 10 minutes
Cooking time: 7 minutes
Servings: 4

Ingredients:
- 8 pork sausage links, sliced
- 1 pound mixed cherry tomatoes, cut in half
- 4 cups baby spinach
- 1 tablespoon avocado oil
- 1 pound mozzarella cheese, cubed
- 2 tablespoons lemon juice
- ⅔ cup basil pesto
- Salt and ground black pepper, to taste

Directions:
Heat up a pan with the oil over medium-high heat, add the sausage slices, stir, and cook them for 4 minutes on each side. In a salad bowl, mix the spinach with mozzarella cheese, tomatoes, salt, pepper, lemon juice, and pesto, and toss to coat. Add the sausage pieces, toss again, and serve.

Nutrition: Calories - 250, Fat - 12, Fiber - 3, Carbs - 8, Protein - 18

Sausage and Peppers Soup

Preparation time: 10 minutes
Cooking time: 1 hour and 10 minutes
Servings: 6

Ingredients:
- 1 tablespoon avocado oil
- 32 ounces pork sausage meat
- 10 ounces canned tomatoes, and jalapeños, chopped
- 10 ounces spinach
- 1 green bell pepper, seeded and chopped
- 4 cups beef stock
- 1 teaspoon onion powder
- Salt and ground black pepper, to taste
- 1 tablespoon cumin
- 1 tablespoon chili powder
- 1 teaspoon garlic powder
- 1 teaspoon Italian seasoning

Directions:
Heat up a pot with the oil over medium heat, add the sausage, stir, and brown for a couple of minutes on all sides. Add the green bell pepper, salt, and pepper, stir, and cook for 3 minutes. Add the tomatoes and jalapeños, stir, and cook for 2 minutes. Add the spinach, stir, cover, and cook for 7 minutes. Add the stock, onion powder, garlic powder, chili powder, cumin, salt, pepper, and Italian seasoning, stir, cover the pot, and cook for 30 minutes. Uncover the pot and cook soup for 15 minutes. Divide into bowls and serve.

Nutrition: Calories - 524, Fat - 43, Fiber - 2, Carbs - 4, Protein - 26

Italian Sausage Soup

Preparation time: 10 minutes
Cooking time: 30 minutes
Servings: 12

Ingredients:
- ½ gallon chicken stock
- A drizzle of avocado oil
- 1 cup heavy cream
- 10 ounces spinach
- 6 bacon slices, chopped
- 1 pound radishes, chopped
- 2 garlic cloves, peeled and minced
- Salt and ground black pepper, to taste
- A pinch of red pepper flakes
- 1 onion, peeled and chopped
- 1½ pounds hot pork sausage, chopped

Directions:
Heat up a pot with a drizzle of avocado oil over medium-high heat, add the sausage, onion, and garlic, stir, and brown for a few minutes. Add the stock, spinach, and radishes, stir, and bring to a simmer. Add the bacon, cream, salt, pepper, and red pepper flakes, stir, and cook for 20 minutes. Divide into bowls and serve.

Nutrition: Calories - 291, Fat - 22, Fiber - 2, Carbs - 4, Protein - 17

Ketogenic Vegetable Recipes

Puréed Broccoli and Cauliflower

Preparation time: 10 minutes
Cooking time: 15 minutes
Servings: 5

Ingredients:

- 1 cauliflower head, separated into florets
- 1 broccoli head, separated into florets
- Salt and ground black pepper, to taste
- 2 garlic cloves, peeled and minced
- 2 bacon slices, chopped
- 2 tablespoons butter

Directions:
Heat up a pot with the butter over medium-high heat, add the garlic and bacon, stir, and cook for 3 minutes. Add the cauliflower and broccoli florets, stir, and cook for 2 minutes. Add the water to cover them, cover the pot, and simmer for 10 minutes. Add the salt and pepper, stir again, and blend soup using an immersion blender. Simmer for a couple minutes over medium heat, ladle into bowls, and serve.

Nutrition: Calories - 230, Fat - 3, Fiber - 3, Carbs - 6, Protein - 10

Broccoli Stew

Preparation time: 10 minutes
Cooking time: 40 minutes
Servings: 4

Ingredients:

- 1 broccoli head, separated into florets
- 2 teaspoons coriander seeds
- A drizzle of olive oil
- 1 onion, peeled and chopped
- Salt and ground black pepper, to taste
- A pinch of red pepper, crushed
- 1 small ginger piece, peeled, and chopped
- 1 garlic clove, peeled and minced
- 28 ounces canned pureed tomatoes

Directions:
Put water in a pot, add the salt, bring to a boil over medium-high heat, add the broccoli florets, steam them for 2 minutes, transfer them to a bowl filled with ice water, drain them, and leave aside. Heat up a pan over medium-high heat, add the coriander seeds, toast them for 4 minutes, transfer to a grinder, ground them, and set aside as well. Heat up a pot with the oil over medium heat, add the onions, salt, pepper, and red pepper, stir, and cook for 7 minutes. Add the ginger, garlic, and coriander seeds, stir, and cook for 3 minutes. Add the tomatoes, bring to a boil, and simmer for 10 minutes. Add the broccoli, stir and cook the stew for 12 minutes. Divide into bowls and serve.

Nutrition: Calories - 150, Fat - 4, Fiber - 2, Carbs - 5, Protein - 12

Watercress Soup

Preparation time: 10 minutes
Cooking time: 10 minutes
Servings: 4

Ingredients:

- 6 cup chicken stock
- ¼ cup sherry
- 2 teaspoons coconut aminos
- 6, and ½ cups watercress
- Salt and ground black pepper, to taste
- 2 teaspoons sesame seed
- 3 shallots, peeled and chopped
- 3 egg whites, whisked

Directions:
Put the stock into a pot, mix with salt, pepper, sherry, and coconut aminos, stir, and bring to a boil over medium-high heat. Add the shallots, watercress, and egg whites, stir, bring to a boil, divide into bowls, and serve with sesame seeds sprinkled on top.

Nutrition: Calories - 50, Fat - 1, Fiber - 0, Carbs - 1, Protein - 5

Bok Choy Soup

Preparation time: 10 minutes
Cooking time: 15 minutes
Servings: 4

Ingredients:
- 3 cups beef stock
- 1 onion, peeled and chopped
- 1 bunch bok choy, chopped
- 1½ cups mushrooms, chopped
- Salt and ground black pepper, to taste
- ½ tablespoon red pepper flakes
- 3 tablespoons coconut aminos
- 3 tablespoons Parmesan cheese, grated
- 2 tablespoons Worcestershire sauce
- 2 bacon strips, chopped

Directions:
Heat up a pot over medium-high heat, add the bacon, stir, cook until it until crispy, transfer to paper towels, and drain the grease. Heat up the pot again over medium heat, add the mushrooms and onions, stir, and cook for 5 minutes. Add the stock, bok choy, coconut aminos, salt, pepper, pepper flakes, and Worcestershire sauce, stir, cover, and cook until bok choy is tender. Ladle the soup into bowls, sprinkle Parmesan cheese, and bacon, and serve.

Nutrition: Calories - 100, Fat - 3, Fiber - 1, Carbs - 2, Protein - 6

Bok Choy Stir-fry

Preparation time: 10 minutes
Cooking time: 7 minutes
Servings: 2

Ingredients:
- 2 garlic cloves, peeled and minced
- 2 cup bok choy, chopped
- 2 bacon slices, chopped
- Salt and ground black pepper, to taste
- A drizzle of avocado oil

Directions:
Heat up a pan with the oil over medium heat, add the bacon, stir, and brown until crispy, transfer to paper towels, and drain the grease. Return the pan to medium heat, add the garlic and bok choy, stir, and cook for 4 minutes. Add the salt, pepper, and return the bacon to the pan, stir, cook for 1 minute, divide on plates, and serve.

Nutrition: Calories - 50, Fat - 1, Fiber - 1, Carbs - 2, Protein - 2

Cream of Celery Soup

Preparation time: 10 minutes
Cooking time: 40 minutes
Servings: 4

Ingredients:
- 1 bunch celery, chopped
- Salt and ground black pepper, to taste
- 3 bay leaves
- ½ garlic head, peeled, and chopped
- 2 onions, peeled and chopped
- 4 cups chicken stock
- ¾ cup heavy cream
- 2 tablespoons butter

Directions:
Heat up a pot with the butter over medium-high heat, add the onions, salt, and pepper, stir, and cook for 5 minutes. Add the bay leaves, garlic, and celery, stir, and cook for 15 minutes. Add the stock, more salt and pepper, stir, cover the pot, reduce the heat, and simmer for 20 minutes. Add the cream, stir, and blend everything using an immersion blender. Ladle into soup bowls and serve.

Nutrition: Calories - 150, Fat - 3, Fiber - 1, Carbs - 2, Protein - 6

Celery Soup

Preparation time: 10 minutes
Cooking time: 25 minutes
Servings: 8

Ingredients:
- 26 ounces celery leaves, and stalks, chopped
- 1 tablespoon dried onion flakes
- Salt and ground black pepper, to taste
- 3 teaspoons fenugreek powder
- 3 teaspoons vegetable stock powder
- 10 ounces sour cream

Directions:
Put the celery into a pot, add the water to cover, add the onion flakes, salt, pepper, stock powder, and fenugreek powder, stir, bring to a boil over medium heat, and simmer for 20 minutes. Use an immersion blender to make the cream, add the sour cream, more salt and pepper, and blend again. Heat up soup again over medium heat, ladle into bowls, and serve.

Nutrition: Calories - 140, Fat - 2, Fiber - 1, Carbs - 5, Protein - 10

Celery Stew

Preparation time: 10 minutes
Cooking time: 30 minutes
Servings: 6

Ingredients:
- 1 celery bunch, chopped
- 1 onion, peeled and chopped
- 1 bunch green onion, peeled and chopped
- 4 garlic cloves, peeled and minced
- Salt and ground black pepper, to taste
- 1 fresh parsley bunch, chopped
- 2 fresh mint bunches, chopped
- 3 dried Persian lemons, pricked with a fork
- 2 cups water
- 2 teaspoons chicken bouillon
- 4 tablespoons olive oil

Directions:
Heat up a pot with the oil over medium-high heat, add the onion, green onions, and garlic, stir, and cook for 6 minutes. Add the celery, Persian lemons, chicken bouillon, salt, pepper, and water, stir, cover pot, and simmer on medium heat for 20 minutes. Add the parsley and mint, stir, and cook for 10 minutes. Divide into bowls and serve.

Nutrition: Calories - 170, Fat - 7, Fiber - 4, Carbs - 6, Protein - 10

Spinach Soup

Preparation time: 10 minutes
Cooking time: 15 minutes
Servings: 8

Ingredients:
- 2 tablespoons butter
- 20 ounces spinach, chopped
- 1 teaspoon garlic, minced
- Salt and ground black pepper, to taste
- 45 ounces chicken stock
- ½ teaspoon ground nutmeg
- 2 cups heavy cream
- 1 onion, peeled and chopped

Directions:
Heat up a pot with the butter over medium heat, add the onion, stir, and cook for 4 minutes. Add the garlic, stir, and cook for 1 minute. Add the spinach and stock, stir, and cook for 5 minutes. Blend soup with an immersion blender, and heat up the soup again. Add the salt, pepper, nutmeg, and cream, stir, and cook for 5 minutes. Ladle into bowls and serve.

Nutrition: Calories - 245, Fat - 24, Fiber - 3, Carbs - 4, Protein - 6

Sautéed Mustard Greens

Preparation time: 10 minutes
Cooking time: 20 minutes
Servings: 4

Ingredients:
- 2 garlic cloves, peeled and minced
- 1 tablespoon olive oil
- 2½ pounds collard greens, chopped
- 1 teaspoon lemon juice
- 1 tablespoon butter
- Salt and ground black pepper, to taste

Directions:
Put some water in a pot, add the salt, and bring to a simmer over medium heat. Add the greens, cover, and cook for 15 minutes. Drain the collard greens well, press the liquid out, and put them into a bowl. Heat up a pan with the oil and butter over medium-high heat, add the collard greens, salt, pepper, and garlic. Stir well and cook for 5 minutes. Add more salt and pepper if needed, drizzle with lemon juice, stir, divide on plates, and serve.

Nutrition: Calories - 151, Fat - 6, Fiber - 3, Carbs - 7, Protein - 8

Collard Greens and Ham

Preparation time: 10 minutes
Cooking time: 1 hour and 40 minutes
Servings: 4

Ingredients:
- 4 ounces ham, boneless, cooked, and chopped
- 1 tablespoon olive oil
- 2 pounds collard greens, cut in medium strips
- 1 teaspoon red pepper flakes
- Salt and ground black pepper, to taste
- 2 cups chicken stock
- 1 onion, peeled and chopped
- 4 ounces dry white wine
- 1 ounce salt pork
- ¼ cup apple cider vinegar
- ½ cup butter, melted

Directions:
Heat up a pan with the oil over medium-high heat, add the ham and onion, stir, and cook for 4 minutes. Add the salt pork, collard greens, stock, vinegar, and wine, stir, and bring to a boil. Reduce the heat, cover the pan, and cook for 1 hour and 30 minutes, stirring from time to time. Add the butter, discard the salt pork, stir, cook everything for 10 minutes, divide on plates, and serve.

Nutrition: Calories - 150, Fat - 12, Fiber - 2, Carbs - 4, Protein - 8

Collard Greens and Tomatoes

Preparation time: 10 minutes
Cooking time: 12 minutes
Servings: 5

Ingredients:
- 1 pound collard greens
- 3 bacon strips, chopped
- ¼ cup cherry tomatoes, halved
- 1 tablespoon apple cider vinegar
- 2 tablespoons chicken stock
- Salt and ground black pepper, to taste

Directions:
Heat up a pan over medium heat, add the bacon, stir, and cook until it browns. Add the tomatoes, collard greens, vinegar, stock, salt, and pepper, stir, and cook for 8 minutes. Add more salt, and pepper, stir again gently, divide on plates, and serve.

Nutrition: Calories - 120, Fat - 8, Fiber - 1, Carbs - 3, Protein - 7

Sautéed Mustard Greens

Preparation time: 5 minutes
Cooking time: 15 minutes
Servings: 4

Ingredients:
- 2 garlic cloves, peeled and minced
- 1 pound mustard greens, torn
- 1 tablespoon olive oil
- ½ cup onion, sliced
- Salt and ground black pepper, to taste
- 3 tablespoons vegetable stock
- ¼ teaspoon dark sesame oil

Directions:
Heat up a pan with the oil over medium heat, add the onions, stir, and brown them for 10 minutes. Add the garlic, stir, and cook for 1 minute. Add the stock, greens, salt, and pepper, stir, and cook for 5 minutes. Add more salt and pepper, and sesame oil, toss to coat, divide on plates, and serve.

Nutrition: Calories - 120, Fat - 3, Fiber - 1, Carbs - 3, Protein - 6

Collard Greens and Poached Eggs

Preparation time: 10 minutes
Cooking time: 15 minutes
Servings: 6

Ingredients:
- 1 tablespoon chipotle in adobo, mashed
- 6 eggs
- 3 tablespoons butter
- 1 onion, peeled and chopped
- 2 garlic cloves, peeled and minced
- 6 bacon slices, chopped
- 3 bunches collard greens, chopped
- ½ cup chicken stock
- Salt and ground black pepper, to taste
- 1 tablespoon lime juice
- Cheddar cheese, grated, for serving

Directions:
Heat up a pan over medium-high heat, add the bacon, cook until crispy, transfer to paper towels, drain grease, and leave aside. Heat up the pan again over medium heat, add the garlic and onion, stir, and cook for 2 minutes. Return the bacon to the pan, stir, and cook for 3 minutes. Add the chipotle in adobo paste, collard greens, salt, and pepper, stir, and cook for 10 minutes. Add the stock and lime juice, and stir. Make 6 holes in collard greens mixture, divide butter in them, crack an egg in each hole, cover the pan, and cook until eggs are done. Divide this on plates and serve with cheddar cheese sprinkled on top.

Nutrition: Calories - 245, Fat - 20, Fiber - 1, Carbs - 5, Protein - 12

Collard Greens Soup

Preparation time: 10 minutes
Cooking time: 40 minutes
Servings: 12

Ingredients:
- 1 teaspoon chili powder
- 1 tablespoon avocado oil
- 2 teaspoons smoked paprika
- 1 teaspoon cumin
- 1 onion, peeled and chopped
- A pinch of red pepper flakes
- 10 cups water
- 3 celery stalks, chopped
- 3 carrots, peeled and chopped
- 15 ounces canned diced tomatoes
- 2 tablespoons tamari sauce
- 6 ounces canned tomato paste
- 2 tablespoons lemon juice
- Salt and ground black pepper, to taste
- 6 cups collard greens, stems discarded
- 1 tablespoon swerve
- 1 teaspoon dried garlic
- 1 tablespoon herb seasoning

Directions:
Heat up a pot with the oil over medium-high heat, add the cumin, pepper flakes, paprika, and chili powder, and stir well. Add the celery, onion, and carrots, stir, and cook for 10 minutes. Add the tamari sauce, tomatoes, tomato paste, water, lemon juice, salt, pepper, herb seasoning, swerve, garlic granules, and collard greens, stir, bring to a boil, cover, and cook for 30 minutes. Stir again, ladle into bowls, and serve.

Nutrition: Calories - 150, Fat - 3, Fiber - 2, Carbs - 4, Protein – 8

Spring Greens Soup

Preparation time: 10 minutes
Cooking time: 30 minutes
Servings: 4

Ingredients:
- 2 cups mustard greens, chopped
- 2 cups collard greens, chopped
- 3 quarts vegetable stock
- 1 onion, peeled and chopped
- Salt and ground black pepper, to taste
- 2 tablespoons coconut aminos
- 2 teaspoons fresh ginger, grated

Directions:
Put the stock into a pot, and bring to a simmer over medium-high heat. Add the mustard, collard greens, onion, salt, pepper, coconut aminos, and ginger, stir, cover the pot, and cook for 30 minutes. Blend the soup using an immersion blender, add more salt, and pepper, heat up over medium heat, ladle into soup bowls, and serve.

Nutrition: Calories - 140, Fat - 2, Fiber - 1, Carbs - 3, Protein - 7

Mustard Greens and Spinach Soup

Preparation time: 10 minutes
Cooking time: 15 minutes
Servings: 6

Ingredients:
- ½ teaspoon fenugreek seeds
- 1 teaspoon cumin seeds
- 1 tablespoon avocado oil
- 1 teaspoon coriander seeds
- 1 cup onion, chopped
- 1 tablespoon garlic, minced
- 1 tablespoon fresh ginger, grated
- ½ teaspoon turmeric
- 5 cups mustard greens, chopped
- 3 cups coconut milk
- 1 tablespoon jalapeño, chopped
- 5 cups spinach, torn
- Salt and ground black pepper, to taste
- 2 teaspoons butter
- ½ teaspoon paprika

Directions:
Heat up a pot with the oil over medium-high heat, add the coriander, fenugreek, and cumin seeds, stir, and brown them for 2 minutes. Add the onions, stir, and cook for 3 minutes. Add the half of the garlic, jalapeños, ginger, and turmeric, stir, and cook for 3 minutes. Add the mustard greens, and spinach, stir, and sauté everything for 10 minutes. Add the milk, salt, and pepper, and blend the soup using an immersion blender. Heat up a pan with the butter over medium heat, add the garlic, and paprika, stir well, and take off the heat. Heat up the soup over medium heat, ladle into soup bowls, drizzle with butter and sprinkle with paprika all over, and serve.

Nutrition: Calories - 143, Fat - 6, Fiber - 3, Carbs - 7, Protein - 7

Roasted Asparagus

Preparation time: 10 minutes
Cooking time: 10 minutes
Servings: 3

Ingredients:
- 1 asparagus bunch, trimmed
- 3 teaspoons avocado oil
- A splash of lemon juice
- Salt and ground black pepper, to taste
- 1 tablespoon fresh oregano, chopped

Directions:
Spread the asparagus spears on a lined baking sheet, season with salt, and pepper, drizzle with oil and lemon juice, sprinkle with oregano, and toss to coat well. Place in an oven at 425°F, and bake for 10 minutes. Divide on plates and serve.

Nutrition: Calories - 130, Fat - 1, Fiber - 1, Carbs - 2, Protein - 3

Asparagus Fries

Preparation time: 10 minutes
Cooking time: 10 minutes
Servings: 2

Ingredients:
- ¼ cup Parmesan cheese, grated
- 16 asparagus spears, trimmed
- 1 egg, whisked
- ½ teaspoon onion powder
- 2 ounces pork rinds

Directions:
Crush the pork rinds, and put them in a bowl. Add the onion powder and cheese, and stir. Roll the asparagus spears in egg, then dip them in pork rind mixture, and arrange them all on a lined baking sheet. Place in an oven at 425°F and bake for 10 minutes. Divide on plates and serve them with some sour cream on the side.

Nutrition: Calories - 120, Fat - 2, Fiber - 2, Carbs - 5, Protein - 8

Asparagus and Browned Butter

Preparation time: 10 minutes
Cooking time: 15 minutes
Servings: 4

Ingredients:
- 5 ounces butter
- 1 tablespoon avocado oil
- 1½ pounds asparagus, trimmed
- 1½ tablespoons lemon juice
- A pinch of cayenne pepper
- 8 tablespoons sour cream
- Salt and ground black pepper, to taste
- 3 ounces Parmesan cheese, grated
- 4 eggs

Directions:
Heat up a pan with 2 ounces butter over medium-high heat, add the eggs, some salt and pepper, stir, and scramble them. Transfer the eggs to a blender, add the Parmesan cheese, sour cream, salt, pepper, and cayenne pepper, and blend everything well. Heat up a pan with the oil over medium-high heat, add the asparagus, salt, and pepper, roast for a few minutes, transfer to a plate, and set aside. Heat up the pan again with the rest of the butter over medium-high heat, stir until brown, take off the heat, add the lemon juice, and stir well. Heat up the butter again, return the asparagus to the pan, toss to coat, heat up well, and divide on plates. Add the blended eggs on top and serve.

Nutrition: Calories - 160, Fat - 7, Fiber - 2, Carbs - 6, Protein - 10

Asparagus Frittata

Preparation time: 10 minutes
Cooking time: 15 minutes
Servings: 4

Ingredients:
- ¼ cup onion, chopped
- A drizzle of olive oil
- 1 pound asparagus spears, cut into 1-inch pieces
- Salt and ground black pepper, to taste
- 4 eggs, whisked
- 1 cup cheddar cheese, grated

Directions:
Heat up a pan with the oil over medium-high heat, add the onions, stir, and cook for 3 minutes. Add the asparagus, stir, and cook for 6 minutes. Add the eggs, stir, and cook for 3 minutes. Add the salt and pepper, sprinkle with the cheese, place in an oven, and broil for 3 minutes. Divide the frittata on plates and serve.

Nutrition: Calories - 200, Fat - 12, Fiber - 2, Carbs - 5, Protein - 14

Creamy Asparagus

Preparation time: 10 minutes
Cooking time: 15 minutes
Servings: 3

Ingredients:
- 10 ounces asparagus spears, cut into medium-sized pieces, and steamed
- Salt and ground black pepper, to taste
- 2 tablespoons Parmesan cheese, grated
- ⅓ cup Monterey jack cheese, shredded
- 2 tablespoons mustard
- 2 ounces cream cheese
- ⅓ cup heavy cream
- 3 tablespoons bacon, cooked and crumbled

Directions:
Heat up a pan with the mustard, heavy cream, and cream cheese over medium heat and stir well. Add the Monterey Jack cheese, and Parmesan cheese, stir, and cook until it melts. Add the half of the bacon, and the asparagus, stir, and cook for 3 minutes. Add the rest of the bacon, plus salt and pepper, stir, cook for 5 minutes, divide on plates, and serve.

Nutrition: Calories - 256, Fat - 23, Fiber - 2, Carbs - 5, Protein - 13

Alfalfa Sprouts Salad

Preparation time: 10 minutes
Cooking time: 0 minutes
Servings: 4

Ingredients:
- 1 green apple, cored, and julienned
- 1½ teaspoons dark sesame oil
- 4 cups alfalfa sprouts
- Salt and ground black pepper, to taste
- 1½ teaspoons grape seed oil
- ¼ cup coconut milk yogurt
- 4 nasturtium leaves

Directions:
In a salad bowl, mix the sprouts with apple and nasturtium. Add the salt, pepper, sesame oil, grape seed oil, and coconut yogurt, toss to coat, and divide on plates, and serve.

Nutrition: Calories - 100, Fat - 3, Fiber - 1, Carbs - 2, Protein - 6

Roasted Radishes

Preparation time: 10 minutes
Cooking time: 35 minutes
Servings: 2

Ingredients:
- 2 cups radishes, cut in quarters
- Salt and ground black pepper, to taste
- 2 tablespoons butter, melted
- 1 tablespoon fresh chives, chopped
- 1 tablespoon lemon zest

Directions:
Spread the radishes on a lined baking sheet. Add the salt, pepper, chives, lemon zest, and butter, toss to coat, and bake in the oven at 375°F for 35 minutes. Divide on plates and serve.

Nutrition: Calories - 122, Fat - 12, Fiber - 1, Carbs - 3, Protein - 14

Radish Hash Browns

Preparation time: 10 minutes
Cooking time: 10 minutes
Servings: 4

Ingredients:
- ½ teaspoon onion powder
- 1 pound radishes, shredded
- ½ teaspoon garlic powder
- Salt and ground black pepper, to taste
- 4 eggs
- ⅓ cup Parmesan cheese, grated

Directions:
In a bowl, mix the radishes with salt, pepper, onion, and garlic powder, eggs, and Parmesan cheese, and stir well. Spread on a lined baking sheet, place in an oven at 375°F, and bake for 10 minutes. Divide the hash browns on plates and serve.

Nutrition: Calories - 80, Fat - 5, Fiber - 2, Carbs - 5, Protein - 7

Crispy Radishes

Preparation time: 10 minutes
Cooking time: 20 minutes
Servings: 4

Ingredients:
- Vegetable oil cooking spray
- 15 radishes, sliced
- Salt and ground black pepper, to taste
- 1 tablespoon fresh chives, chopped

Directions:
Arrange the radish slices on a lined baking sheet and spray them with cooking oil. Season with salt and pepper, sprinkle with the chives, place in an oven at 375°F, and bake for 10 minutes. Flip them and bake for 10 minutes. Serve cold.

Nutrition: Calories - 30, Fat - 1, Fiber - 0. 4, Carbs - 1, Protein - 0. 1

Creamy Radishes

Preparation time: 10 minutes
Cooking time: 25 minutes
Servings: 1

Ingredients:
- 7 ounces radishes, cut in half
- 2 tablespoons sour cream
- 2 bacon slices
- 1 tablespoon green onion, peeled and chopped
- 1 tablespoon cheddar cheese, grated
- Hot sauce, to taste
- Salt and ground black pepper, to taste

Directions:
Put the radishes into a pot, add the water to cover, bring to a boil over medium heat, cook them for 10 minutes, and drain. Heat up a pan over medium-high heat, add the bacon, cook until crispy, transfer to paper towels, drain the grease, crumble, and leave aside. Return the pan to medium heat, add the radishes, stir, and sauté them for 7 minutes. Add the onion, salt, pepper, hot sauce, and sour cream, stir, and cook for 7 minutes. Transfer to a plate, top with crumbled bacon and cheddar cheese, and serve.

Nutrition: Calories - 340, Fat - 23, Fiber - 3, Carbs - 6, Protein - 15

Radish Soup

Preparation time: 10 minutes
Cooking time: 20 minutes
Servings: 4

Ingredients:
- 2 bunches radishes, cut in quarters
- Salt and ground black pepper, to taste
- 6 cups chicken stock
- 2 stalks celery, chopped
- 3 tablespoons coconut oil
- 6 garlic cloves, peeled and minced
- 1 onion, peeled and chopped

Directions:
Heat up a pot with the oil over medium heat, add the onion, celery, and garlic, stir, and cook for 5 minutes. Add the radishes, stock, salt, and pepper, stir, bring to a boil, cover, and simmer for 15 minutes. Divide into soup bowls and serve.

Nutrition: Calories - 120, Fat - 2, Fiber - 1, Carbs - 3, Protein - 10

Avocado Salad

Preparation time: 10 minutes
Cooking time: 0 minutes
Servings: 4

Ingredients:
- 2 avocados, pitted, and mashed
- Salt and ground black pepper, to taste
- ¼ teaspoon lemon stevia
- 1 tablespoon white vinegar
- 14 ounces coleslaw mix
- Juice from 2 limes
- ¼ cup onion, chopped
- ¼ cup fresh cilantro, chopped
- 2 tablespoons olive oil

Directions:
Put the coleslaw mixture in a salad bowl. Add the avocado mash and onions, and toss to coat. In a bowl, mix the lime juice with salt, pepper, oil, vinegar, and stevia, and stir well. Add this to salad, toss to coat, sprinkle cilantro, and serve.

Nutrition: Calories - 100, Fat - 10, Fiber - 2, Carbs - 5, Protein - 8

Avocado and Egg Salad

Preparation time: 10 minutes
Cooking time: 7 minutes
Servings: 4

Ingredients:
- 4 cups mixed lettuce leaves, torn
- 4 eggs
- 1 avocado, pitted, and sliced
- ¼ cup mayonnaise
- 2 teaspoons mustard
- 2 garlic cloves, peeled and minced
- 1 tablespoon fresh chives, chopped
- Salt and ground black pepper, to taste

Directions:
Put water in a pot, add the some salt, add the eggs, bring to a boil over medium-high heat, boil for 7 minutes, drain, cool, peel, and chop them. In a salad bowl, mix the lettuce with eggs, and avocado. Add the chives and garlic, some salt, and pepper, and toss to coat. In a bowl, mix the mustard with mayonnaise, salt, and pepper, and stir well. Add this to the salad, toss well, and serve.

Nutrition: Calories - 234, Fat - 12, Fiber - 4, Carbs - 7, Protein - 12

Avocado and Cucumber Salad

Preparation time: 10 minutes
Cooking time: 0 minutes
Servings: 4

Ingredients:
- 1 onion, peeled and sliced
- 1 cucumber, sliced
- 2 avocados, pitted, peeled, and chopped
- 1 pound cherry tomatoes, halved
- 2 tablespoons olive oil
- ¼ cup fresh cilantro, chopped
- 2 tablespoons lemon juice
- Salt and ground black pepper, to taste

Directions:
In a large salad bowl, mix the tomatoes with the cucumber, onion, and avocado, and stir. Add the oil, salt, pepper, and lemon juice, and toss to coat well. Serve cold with cilantro on top.

Nutrition: Calories - 140, Fat - 4, Fiber - 2, Carbs - 4, Protein - 5

Avocado Soup

Preparation time: 10 minutes
Cooking time: 10 minutes
Servings: 4

Ingredients:
- 2 avocados, pitted, peeled, and chopped
- 3 cups chicken stock
- 2 scallions, chopped
- Salt and ground black pepper, to taste
- 2 tablespoons butter
- ⅔ cup heavy cream

Directions:
Heat up a pot with the butter over medium heat, add the scallions, stir, and cook for 2 minutes. Add the 2 ½ cups stock, stir, and simmer for 3 minutes. In a blender, mix the avocados with the rest of the stock, salt, pepper, and heavy cream, and pulse well. Add this to the pot, stir well, cook for 2 minutes, and season with more salt and pepper. Stir well, ladle into soup bowls, and serve.

Nutrition: Calories - 332, Fat - 23, Fiber - 4, Carbs - 6, Protein - 6

Avocado and Bacon Soup

Preparation time: 10 minutes
Cooking time: 10 minutes
Servings: 4

Ingredients:
- 2 avocados, pitted, and cut in half
- 4 cups chicken stock
- ⅓ cup fresh cilantro, chopped
- Juice of ½ lime
- 1 teaspoon garlic powder
- ½ pound bacon, cooked, and chopped
- Salt and ground black pepper, to taste

Directions:
Put the stock in a pot and bring to a boil over medium-high heat. In a blender, mix the avocados with garlic powder, cilantro, lime juice, salt, and pepper, and blend well. Add this to the stock and blend using an immersion blender. Add the bacon, more salt and pepper, stir, cook for 3 minutes, ladle into soup bowls, and serve.

Nutrition: Calories - 300, Fat - 23, Fiber - 5, Carbs - 6, Protein - 17

Thai Avocado Soup

Preparation time: 10 minutes
Cooking time: 10 minutes
Servings: 4

Ingredients:
- 1 cup coconut milk
- 2 teaspoons Thai green curry paste
- 1 avocado, pitted, peeled, and chopped
- 1 tablespoon fresh cilantro, chopped
- Salt and ground black pepper, to taste
- 2 cups vegetable stock
- Lime wedges, for serving

Directions:
In a blender, mix the avocado with salt, pepper, curry paste, and coconut milk, and pulse well. Transfer this to a pot and heat up over medium heat. Add the stock, stir, bring to a simmer, and cook for 5 minutes. Add the cilantro, more salt and pepper, stir, cook for 1 minute, ladle into soup bowls, and serve with lime wedges.

Nutrition: Calories - 240, Fat - 4, Fiber - 2, Carbs - 6, Protein - 12

Arugula Salad

Preparation time: 10 minutes
Cooking time: 0 minutes
Servings: 4

Ingredients:
- 1 white onion, peeled and chopped
- 1 tablespoon vinegar
- 1 cup hot water
- 1 bunch baby arugula
- ¼ cup walnuts, chopped
- 2 tablespoons fresh cilantro, chopped
- 2 garlic cloves, peeled and minced
- 2 tablespoons olive oil
- Salt and ground black pepper, to taste
- 1 tablespoon lemon juice

Directions:
In a bowl, mix the water with vinegar, add the onion, set aside for 5 minutes, and drain well. In a salad bowl, mix the arugula with the walnuts and onion, and stir. Add the garlic, salt, pepper, lemon juice, cilantro, and oil, toss well, and serve.

Nutrition: Calories - 200, Fat - 2, Fiber - 1, Carbs - 5, Protein - 7

Arugula Soup

Preparation time: 10 minutes
Cooking time: 13 minutes
Servings: 6

Ingredients:
- 1 onion, peeled and chopped
- 1 tablespoon olive oil
- 2 garlic cloves, peeled and minced
- ½ cup coconut milk
- 10 ounces baby arugula
- 2 tablespoons fresh mint, chopped, and
- 2 tablespoons fresh tarragon, chopped
- 2 tablespoons fresh parsley, chopped
- 2 tablespoons fresh chives, chopped
- 4 tablespoons coconut milk yogurt
- 6 cups chicken stock
- Salt and ground black pepper, to taste

Directions:
Heat up a pot with the oil over medium-high heat, add the onion and garlic, stir, and cook for 5 minutes. Add the stock, and milk, stir, and bring to a simmer. Add the arugula, tarragon, parsley, and mint, stir, and cook for 6 minutes. Add the coconut yogurt, salt, pepper, and chives, stir, cook for 2 minutes, divide into soup bowls, and serve.

Nutrition: Calories - 200, Fat - 4, Fiber - 2, Carbs - 6, Protein - 10

Arugula and Broccoli Soup

Preparation time: 10 minutes
Cooking time: 20 minutes
Servings: 4

Ingredients:
- 1 onion, peeled and chopped
- 1 tablespoon olive oil
- 1 garlic clove, peeled and minced
- 1 broccoli head, separated into florets
- Salt and ground black pepper, to taste
- 2, and ½ cups vegetable stock
- 1 teaspoon cumin
- Juice of ½ lemon
- 1 cup arugula leaves

Directions:
Heat up a pot with the oil over medium-high heat, add the onions, stir, and cook for 4 minutes. Add the garlic, stir, and cook for 1 minute. Add the broccoli, cumin, salt, and pepper, stir, and cook for 4 minutes. Add the stock, stir, and cook for 8 minutes. Blend the soup using an immersion blender, add half of the arugula, and blend again. Add the rest of the arugula, stir, and heat up the soup again. Add the lemon juice, stir, ladle into soup bowls, and serve.

Nutrition: Calories - 150, Fat - 3, Fiber - 1, Carbs - 3, Protein - 7

Zucchini Cream

Preparation time: 10 minutes
Cooking time: 25 minutes
Servings: 8

Ingredients:
- 6 zucchini, cut in half and sliced
- Salt and ground black pepper, to taste
- 1 tablespoon butter
- 28 ounces vegetable stock
- 1 teaspoon dried oregano
- ½ cup onion, chopped
- 3 garlic cloves, peeled and minced
- 2 ounces Parmesan cheese, grated
- ¾ cup heavy cream

Directions:
Heat up a pot with the butter over medium-high heat, add the onion, stir, and cook for 4 minutes. Add the garlic, stir, and cook for 2 minutes. Add the zucchini, stir, and cook for 3 minutes. Add the stock, stir, bring to a boil, and simmer over medium heat for 15 minutes. Add the oregano, salt, and pepper, stir, take off the heat, and blend using an immersion blender. Heat the soup again, add the heavy cream, stir, and bring to a simmer. Add the Parmesan cheese, stir, take off the heat, ladle into bowls, and serve.

Nutrition: Calories - 160, Fat - 4, Fiber - 2, Carbs - 4, Protein - 8

Zucchini and Avocado Soup

Preparation time: 10 minutes
Cooking time: 15 minutes
Servings: 4

Ingredients:
- 1 big avocado, pitted, peeled, and chopped
- 4 scallions, chopped
- 1 teaspoon fresh ginger, grated
- 2 tablespoons avocado oil
- Salt and ground black pepper, to taste
- 2 zucchini, chopped
- 29 ounces vegetable stock
- 1 garlic clove, peeled and minced
- 1 cup water
- 1 tablespoon lemon juice
- 1 red bell pepper, seeded and chopped

Directions:
Heat up a pot with the oil over medium heat, add the onions, stir, and cook for 3 minutes. Add the garlic and ginger, stir, and cook for 1 minute. Add the zucchini, salt, pepper, water, and stock, stir, bring to a boil, cover the pot, and cook for 10 minutes. Take off heat, set the soup aside for a couple of minutes, add the avocado, stir, blend everything using an immersion blender, and heat up again. Add more salt and pepper, plus the bell pepper and lemon juice, stir, heat up soup again, ladle into soup bowls, and serve.

Nutrition: Calories - 154, Fat - 12, Fiber - 3, Carbs - 5, Protein - 4

Swiss Chard Pie

Preparation time: 10 minutes
Cooking time: 45 minutes
Servings: 12

Ingredients:
- 8 cups Swiss chard, chopped
- ½ cup onion, peeled and chopped
- 1 tablespoon olive oil
- 1 garlic clove, peeled and minced
- Salt and ground black pepper, to taste
- 3 eggs
- 2 cups ricotta cheese
- 1 cup mozzarella cheese, shredded
- A pinch of nutmeg
- ¼ cup Parmesan cheese, grated
- 1 pound sausage, chopped

Directions:
Heat up a pan with the oil over medium heat, add the onions and garlic, stir, and cook for 3 minutes. Add the Swiss chard, stir, and cook for 5 minutes. Add the salt, pepper, and nutmeg, stir, take off the heat, and set aside for a few minutes. In a bowl, whisk the eggs with cheeses and stir well. Add the Swiss chard mixture and stir well. Spread the sausage meat on the bottom of a pie pan and press well. Add the Swiss chard, and eggs mixture, spread well, place in an oven at 350°F, and bake for 35 minutes. Set the pie aside to cool down, slice, and serve it.

Nutrition: Calories - 332, Fat - 23, Fiber - 3, Carbs - 4, Protein - 23

Swiss Chard Salad

Preparation time: 10 minutes
Cooking time: 20 minutes
Servings: 4

Ingredients:
- 1 bunch Swiss chard, cut into strips
- 2 tablespoons avocado oil
- 1 onion, peeled and chopped
- A pinch of red pepper flakes
- ¼ cup pine nuts, toasted
- ¼ cup raisins
- 1 tablespoon balsamic vinegar
- Salt and ground black pepper, to taste

Directions:
Heat up a pan with the oil over medium heat, add the chard and onions, stir, and cook for 5 minutes.
Add the salt, pepper, and pepper flakes, stir, and cook for 3 minutes. Put the raisins in a bowl, add the water to cover them, heat them up in a microwave for 1 minute, set aside for 5 minutes, and drain them well. Add the raisins, and pine nuts to the pan with the vinegar, stir, cook for 3 minutes, divide on plates, and serve.

Nutrition: Calories - 120, Fat - 2, Fiber - 1, Carbs - 4, Protein - 8

Green Salad

Preparation time: 10 minutes
Cooking time: 0 minutes
Servings: 4

Ingredients:
- 24 green grapes, halved
- 1 bunch Swiss chard, chopped
- 1 avocado, pitted, peeled, and cubed
- Salt and ground black pepper, to taste
- 2 tablespoons avocado oil
- 1 tablespoon mustard
- 7 sage leaves, chopped
- 1 garlic clove, peeled and minced

Directions:
In a salad bowl, mix the Swiss chard with the grapes and avocado cubes. In a bowl, mix the mustard with the oil, sage, garlic, salt, and pepper, and whisk. Add this to the salad, toss to coat well, and serve.

Nutrition: Calories - 120, Fat - 2, Fiber - 1, Carbs - 4, Protein - 5

Catalan-style Greens

Preparation time: 10 minutes
Cooking time: 15 minutes
Servings: 4

Ingredients:
- 1 apple, cored and chopped
- 1 onion, peeled and sliced
- 3 tablespoons avocado oil
- ¼ cup raisins
- 6 garlic cloves, peeled and chopped
- ¼ cup pine nuts, toasted
- ¼ cup balsamic vinegar
- 2½ cups Swiss chard
- 2½ cups spinach, and
- Salt and ground black pepper, to taste
- A pinch of nutmeg

Directions:
Heat up a pan with the oil over medium-high heat, add the onion, stir, and cook for 3 minutes. Add the apple, stir, and cook for 4 minutes. Add the garlic, stir, and cook for 1 minute. Add the raisins, vinegar, spinach, and chard, stir, and cook for 5 minutes. Add the nutmeg, salt, and pepper, stir, cook for a few seconds, divide on plates, and serve.

Nutrition: Calories - 120, Fat - 1, Fiber - 2, Carbs - 3, Protein - 6

Swiss Chard and Chicken Soup

Preparation time: 10 minutes
Cooking time: 35 minutes
Servings: 12

Ingredients:
- 4 cups Swiss chard, chopped
- 4 cups chicken breast, cooked, and shredded
- 2 cups water
- 1 cup mushrooms, sliced
- 1 tablespoon garlic, minced
- 1 tablespoon coconut oil, melted
- ¼ cup onion, peeled and chopped
- 8 cups chicken stock
- 2 cups yellow squash, chopped
- 1 cup green beans, cut into medium-sized pieces
- 2 tablespoons vinegar
- ¼ cup fresh basil, chopped
- Salt and ground black pepper, to taste
- 4 bacon slices, chopped
- ¼ cup sundried tomatoes, cored and chopped

Directions:
Heat up a pot with the oil over medium-high heat, add the bacon, stir, and cook for 2 minutes. Add the tomatoes, garlic, onions, and mushrooms, stir, and cook for 5 minutes. Add the water, stock, and chicken, stir, and cook for 15 minutes. Add the Swiss chard, green beans, squash, salt, and pepper, stir, and cook for 10 minutes. Add the vinegar, basil, salt, and pepper, stir, ladle into soup bowls, and serve.

Nutrition: Calories - 140, Fat - 4, Fiber - 2, Carbs - 4, Protein - 18

Swiss Chard and Vegetable Soup

Preparation time: 10 minutes
Cooking time: 2 hours and 10 minutes
Servings: 4

Ingredients:
- 1 onion, peeled and chopped
- 1 bunch Swiss chard, chopped
- 1 yellow squash, chopped
- 1 zucchini, chopped
- 1 green bell pepper, seeded and chopped
- Salt and ground black pepper, to taste
- 6 carrots, peeled and chopped
- 4 cups tomatoes, cored and chopped
- 1 cup cauliflower florets, chopped
- 1 cup green beans, chopped
- 6 cups chicken stock
- 7 ounces canned tomato paste
- 2 cups water
- 1 pound sausage, chopped
- 2 garlic cloves, peeled and minced
- 2 teaspoons thyme, chopped
- 1 teaspoon dried rosemary
- 1 tablespoon fennel, minced
- ½ teaspoon red pepper flakes
- Some grated Parmesan cheese, for serving

Directions:
Heat up a pan over medium-high heat, add the sausage and garlic, stir and cook until it browns, and transfer along with its juices to a slow cooker. Add the onion, Swiss chard, squash, bell pepper, zucchini, carrots, tomatoes, cauliflower, green beans, tomato paste, stock, water, thyme, fennel, rosemary, pepper flakes, salt, and pepper, stir, cover, and cook on high for 2 hours. Uncover the slow cooker, stir the soup, ladle into bowls, sprinkle Parmesan cheese on top, and serve.

Nutrition: Calories - 150, Fat - 8, Fiber - 2, Carbs - 4, Protein - 9

Roasted Tomato Cream

Preparation time: 10 minutes
Cooking time: 1 hour
Servings: 8

Ingredients:
- 1 jalapeño pepper, chopped
- 4 garlic cloves, peeled and minced
- 2 pounds cherry tomatoes, cut in half
- 1 onion, peeled and cut into wedges
- Salt and ground black pepper, to taste
- ¼ cup olive oil
- ½ teaspoon dried oregano
- 4 cups chicken stock
- ¼ cup fresh basil, chopped
- ½ cup Parmesan cheese, grated

Directions:
Spread the tomatoes, and onion in a baking dish. Add the garlic and chili pepper, season with salt, pepper, and oregano, and drizzle the oil. Toss to coat and bake in the oven at 425°F for 30 minutes. Take the tomato mixture out of the oven, transfer to a pot, add the stock, and heat everything up over medium-high heat. Bring to a boil, cover the pot, reduce heat, and simmer for 20 minutes. Blend using an immersion blender, add the salt and pepper to taste, and basil, stir, and ladle into soup bowls. Sprinkle with Parmesan cheese on top and serve.

Nutrition: Calories - 140, Fat - 2, Fiber - 2, Carbs - 5, Protein - 8

Eggplant Soup

Preparation time: 10 minutes
Cooking time: 50 minutes
Servings: 4

Ingredients:
- 4 tomatoes
- 1 teaspoon garlic, minced
- ¼ onion, peeled and chopped
- Salt and ground black pepper, to taste
- 2 cups chicken stock
- 1 bay leaf
- ½ cup heavy cream
- 2 tablespoons fresh basil, chopped
- 4 tablespoons Parmesan cheese, grated
- 1 tablespoon olive oil
- 1 eggplant, chopped

Directions:
Spread the eggplant pieces on a baking sheet, mix with oil, onion, garlic, salt, and pepper, place in an oven at 400°F, and bake for 15 minutes. Put water in a pot, bring to a boil over medium heat, add the tomatoes, steam them for 1 minute, peel them, and chop. Take the eggplant mixture out of the oven, and transfer to a pot. Add the tomatoes, stock, bay leaf, salt, and pepper, stir, bring to a boil, and simmer for 30 minutes. Add the heavy cream, basil, and Parmesan cheese, stir, ladle into soup bowls, and serve.

Nutrition: Calories - 180, Fat - 2, Fiber - 3, Carbs - 5, Protein - 10

Eggplant Stew

Preparation time: 10 minutes
Cooking time: 30 minutes
Servings: 4

Ingredients:
- 1 onion, peeled and chopped
- 2 garlic cloves, peeled and chopped
- 1 bunch fresh parsley, chopped
- Salt and ground black pepper, to taste
- 1 teaspoon dried oregano
- 2 eggplants, cut into medium-sized chunks
- 2 tablespoons olive oil
- 2 tablespoons capers, chopped
- 12 green olives, pitted and sliced
- 5 tomatoes, cored and chopped
- 3 tablespoons herb vinegar

Directions:
Heat up a pot with the oil over medium heat, add the eggplant, oregano, salt, and pepper, stir, and cook for 5 minutes. Add the garlic, onion, and parsley, stir, and cook for 4 minutes. Add the capers, olives, vinegar, and tomatoes, stir, and cook for 15 minutes. Add more salt and pepper, if needed, stir, divide into bowls, and serve.

Nutrition: Calories - 200, Fat - 13, Fiber - 3, Carbs - 5, Protein - 7

Roasted Bell Peppers Soup

Preparation time: 10 minutes
Cooking time: 15 minutes
Servings: 6

Ingredients:
- 12 ounces roasted bell peppers, seeded and chopped
- 2 tablespoons olive oil
- 2 garlic cloves, peeled and minced
- 29 ounces canned chicken stock
- Salt and ground black pepper, to taste
- 7 ounces water
- ⅔ cup heavy cream
- 1 onion, peeled and chopped
- ¼ cup Parmesan cheese, grated
- 2 celery stalks, chopped

Directions:
Heat up a pot with the oil over medium heat, add the onion, garlic, celery, and some salt, and pepper, stir, and cook for 8 minutes. Add the bell peppers, water, and stock, stir, bring to a boil, cover, reduce the heat, and simmer for 5 minutes. Use an immersion blender to puree the soup, then add more salt, pepper, and cream, stir, bring to a boil, and take off the heat. Ladle into bowls, sprinkle Parmesan cheese, and serve.

Nutrition: Calories - 176, Fat - 13, Fiber - 1, Carbs - 4, Protein - 6

Cabbage Soup

Preparation time: 10 minutes
Cooking time: 45 minutes
Servings: 8

Ingredients:
- 1 garlic clove, peeled and minced
- 1 cabbage head, chopped
- 2 pounds ground beef
- 1 onion, peeled and chopped
- 1 teaspoon cumin
- 4 bouillon cubes
- Salt and ground black pepper, to taste
- 10 ounces canned tomatoes, and green chilies
- 4 cups water

Directions:
Heat up a pan over medium heat, add the beef, stir, and brown for a few minutes. Add the onion, stir, cook for 4 minutes, and transfer to a pot. Heat the pot, add the cabbage, cumin, garlic, bouillon cubes, tomatoes, and chilies, and water, stir, bring to a boil over high heat, cover, reduce temperature, and cook for 40 minutes. Season with salt and pepper, stir, ladle into soup bowls, and serve.

Nutrition: Calories - 200, Fat - 3, Fiber - 2, Carbs - 6, Protein - 8

Ketogenic Dessert Recipes

Chocolate Truffles

Preparation time: 10 minutes
Cooking time: 6 minutes
Servings: 22

Ingredients:
- 1 cup sugar-free chocolate chips
- 2 tablespoons butter
- ⅔ cup heavy cream
- 2 teaspoons brandy
- 2 tablespoons swerve
- ¼ teaspoon vanilla extract
- Cocoa powder

Directions:
Put the heavy cream in a heatproof bowl, add the swerve, butter, and chocolate chips, stir, introduce in a microwave, and heat up for 1 minute. Set aside for 5 minutes, stir well, and mix with brandy, and vanilla extract. Stir again and set aside in the refrigerator for a couple of hours. Use a melon baller to shape the truffles, roll them in cocoa powder, and serve.

Nutrition: Calories - 60, Fat - 5, Fiber - 4, Carbs - 6, Protein - 1

Doughnuts

Preparation time: 10 minutes
Cooking time: 15 minutes
Servings: 24

Ingredients:
- ¼ cup erythritol
- ¼ cup flaxseed meal
- ¾ cup almond flour
- 1 teaspoon baking powder
- 1 teaspoon vanilla extract
- 2 eggs
- 3 tablespoons coconut oil
- ¼ cup coconut milk
- 20 drops red food coloring
- A pinch of salt
- 1 tablespoon cocoa powder

Directions:
In a bowl, mix the flaxseed meal with almond flour, cocoa powder, baking powder, erythritol, and salt, and stir. In another bowl, mix the coconut oil with coconut milk, vanilla extract, food coloring, and eggs, and stir. Combine the 2 mixtures, stir using a hand mixer, transfer to a bag, make a hole in the bag, and shape 12 doughnuts on a baking sheet. Place in an oven at 350°F, and bake for 15 minutes. Arrange them on a platter and serve.

Nutrition: Calories - 60, Fat - 4, Fiber - 0, Carbs - 1, Protein - 2

Chocolate Bombs

Preparation time: 10 minutes
Cooking time: 10 minutes
Servings: 12

Ingredients:
- 10 tablespoons coconut oil
- 3 tablespoons macadamia nuts, chopped
- 2 packets stevia
- 5 tablespoons unsweetened coconut powder
- A pinch of salt

Directions:
Put the coconut oil in a pot and melt over medium heat. Add the stevia, salt, and cocoa powder, stir well, and take off the heat. Spoon this into a candy tray and keep in the refrigerator for a couple of hours. Sprinkle the macadamia nuts on top, and keep in the refrigerator until ready to serve.

Nutrition: Calories - 50, Fat - 1, Fiber - 0, Carbs - 1, Protein - 2

Gelatin

Preparation time: 2 hours 10 minutes
Cooking time: 5 minutes
Servings: 12

Ingredients:
- 2 ounces packets sugar-free gelatin
- 1 cup cold water
- 1 cup hot water
- 3 tablespoons erythritol
- 2 tablespoons gelatin powder
- 1 teaspoon vanilla extract
- 1 cup heavy cream
- 1 cup boiling water

Directions:
Put the gelatin packets in a bowl, add the 1 cup hot water, stir until it dissolves, and then mix with 1 cup cold water. Pour this into a lined square dish, and keep in the refrigerator for 1 hour. Cut into cubes, and set aside. In a bowl, mix the erythritol with vanilla extract, 1 cup boiling water, gelatin, and heavy cream, and stir well. Pour half of this mix into a silicon round mold, spread the gelatin cubes, and then top with the rest of the gelatin. Keep in the refrigerator for 1 more hour and then serve.

Nutrition: Calories - 70, Fat - 1, Fiber - 0, Carbs - 1, Protein - 2

Strawberry Pie

Preparation time: 2 hours and 10 minutes
Cooking time: 5 minutes
Servings: 12

Ingredients:
For the crust:
- 1 cup coconut, shredded
- 1 cup sunflower seeds
- ¼ cup butter
- A pinch of salt

For the filling:
- 1 teaspoon gelatin
- 8 ounces cream cheese
- 4 ounces strawberries
- 2 tablespoons water
- ½ tablespoon lemon juice
- ¼ teaspoon stevia
- ½ cup heavy cream
- 8 ounces strawberries, hulled, and chopped, for serving
- 16 ounces heavy cream, for serving

Directions:
In a food processor, mix the sunflower seeds with coconut, a pinch of salt, and butter, and stir well. Put this into a greased springform pan and press well on the bottom. Heat up a pan with the water over medium heat, add the gelatin, stir until it dissolves, take off the heat, and set aside to cool down. Add this to a food processor, mix with 4 ounces strawberries, cream cheese, lemon juice, and stevia, and blend well. Add the ½ cup heavy cream, stir well, and spread this over the crust. Top with 8 ounces strawberries, and 16 ounces heavy cream, and keep in the refrigerator for 2 hours before slicing and serving.

Nutrition: Calories - 234, Fat - 23, Fiber - 2, Carbs - 6, Protein - 7

Chocolate Pie

Preparation time: 3 hours 10 minutes
Cooking time: 20 minutes
Servings: 10

Ingredients:
For the crust:
- ½ teaspoon baking powder
- 1½ cup almond crust
- A pinch of salt
- ⅓ cup stevia
- 1 egg
- 1½ teaspoons vanilla extract
- 3 tablespoons butter
- 1 teaspoon butter for the pan

For the filling:
- 1 tablespoon vanilla extract
- 4 tablespoons butter
- 4 tablespoons sour cream
- 16 ounces cream cheese
- ½ cup cut stevia
- ½ cup cocoa powder
- 2 teaspoons granulated stevia
- 1 cup whipping cream
- 1 teaspoon vanilla extract

Directions:
Grease a springform pan with 1 teaspoon butter, and set aside. In a bowl, mix the baking powder with ⅓ cup stevia, a pinch of salt and almond flour, and stir. Add the 3 tablespoons butter, egg, and 1½ teaspoon vanilla extract, stir until you obtain a dough. Press this well into springform pan, place in an oven at 375°F, and bake for 11 minutes. Take the pie crust out of the oven, cover with aluminum foil, and bake for 8 minutes. Take it out of the oven and set aside to cool down. In a bowl, mix the cream cheese with 4 tablespoons butter, sour cream, 1 tablespoon vanilla extract, cocoa powder, and ½ cup stevia, and stir well. In another bowl, mix the whipping cream with 2 teaspoons stevia, and 1 teaspoon vanilla extract, and stir using a mixer. Combine the 2 mixtures, pour into pie crust, spread well, place in the refrigerator for 3 hours, and then serve.

Nutrition: Calories - 450, Fat - 43, Fiber - 3, Carbs - 7, Protein - 7

Mini Cheesecakes

Preparation time: 10 minutes
Cooking time: 15 minutes
Servings: 9

Ingredients:
For the cheesecakes:
- 2 tablespoons butter
- 8 ounces cream cheese
- 3 tablespoons coffee
- 3 eggs
- ⅓ cup swerve
- 1 tablespoon sugar-free caramel syrup

For the frosting:
- 3 tablespoons sugar-free caramel syrup
- 3 tablespoons butter
- 8 ounces mascarpone cheese, softened
- 2 tablespoons swerve

Directions:
In a blender, mix the cream cheese with eggs, 2 tablespoons butter, coffee, 1 tablespoon caramel syrup, and ⅓ cup swerve, and pulse well. Spoon this into a cupcakes pan, place in an oven at 350°F, and bake for 15 minutes. Set aside to cool down, and then keep in the freezer for 3 hours. In a bowl, mix the 3 tablespoons butter with 3 tablespoons caramel syrup, 2 tablespoons swerve, and mascarpone cheese, and blend well. Spoon this over cheesecakes and serve.

Nutrition: Calories - 254, Fat - 23, Fiber - 0, Carbs - 1, Protein - 5

Raspberry and Coconut Dessert

Preparation time: 10 minutes
Cooking time: 5 minutes
Servings: 12

Ingredients:
- ½ cup coconut butter
- ½ cup coconut oil
- ½ cup raspberries, dried
- ¼ cup swerve
- ½ cup coconut, shredded

Directions:
In a food processor, blend the dried berries well. Heat up a pan with the butter over medium heat. Add the oil, coconut, and swerve, stir, and cook for 5 minutes. Pour half of this into a lined baking pan and spread well. Add the raspberry powder and spread well. Top with the rest of the butter mixture, spread, and keep in the refrigerator for a couple of hours, then cut into pieces and serve.

Nutrition: Calories - 234, Fat - 22, Fiber - 2, Carbs - 4, Protein - 2

Chocolate Cups

Preparation time: 30 minutes
Cooking time: 5 minutes
Servings: 20

Ingredients:
- ½ cup coconut butter
- ½ cup coconut oil
- 3 tablespoons swerve
- ½ cup coconut, shredded
- 1.5 ounces cocoa butter
- 1 ounces chocolate, unsweetened
- ¼ cup cocoa powder
- ¼ teaspoon vanilla extract
- ¼ cup swerve

Directions:
In a pan, mix the coconut butter with coconut oil, stir, and heat up over medium heat. Add the coconut and 3 tablespoons swerve, stir well, take off the heat, scoop into a lined muffins pan, and keep in the refrigerator for 30 minutes. In a bowl, mix the cocoa butter with the chocolate, vanilla extract, ¼ cup swerve, and stir well. Place this over a bowl filled with boiling water and stir until everything is smooth. Spoon this over coconut cupcakes, keep in the refrigerator for 15 minutes, and then serve.

Nutrition: Calories - 240, Fat - 23, Fiber - 4, Carbs - 5, Protein - 2

Berry Mousse

Preparation time: 10 minutes
Cooking time: 0 minutes
Servings: 12

Ingredients:
- 8 ounces mascarpone cheese
- ¾ teaspoon stevia
- ½ teaspoon vanilla extract
- 1 cup whipping cream
- ½ pint blueberries
- ½ pint strawberries

Directions:
In a bowl, mix the whipping cream with stevia, and mascarpone, and blend well using a mixer. Arrange a layer of blueberries and strawberries in 12 glasses, then a layer of cream, and so on. Serve cold.

Nutrition: Calories - 143, Fat - 12, Fiber - 1, Carbs - 3, Protein - 2

Peanut Butter Fudge

ours and 10 minutes
utes

Ingredients:
- 1 cup peanut butter, unsweetened
- ¼ cup almond milk
- ½ teaspoon vanilla extract
- 2 teaspoons stevia
- 1 cup coconut oil
- A pinch of salt

For the topping:
- 2 tablespoons swerve
- 2 tablespoons melted coconut oil
- ¼ cup cocoa powder

Directions:
In a heatproof bowl, mix the peanut butter with 1 cup coconut oil, stir, and heat up in a microwave until it melts. Add a pinch of salt, almond milk, and stevia, stir well, and pour into a lined loaf pan. Keep in the refrigerator for 2 hours and then slice it. In a bowl, mix the 2 tablespoons melted coconut oil with cocoa powder, and swerve, and stir well. Drizzle the sauce over the peanut butter fudge and serve.

Nutrition: Calories - 265, Fat - 23, Fiber - 2, Carbs - 4, Protein - 6

Lemon Mousse

Preparation time: 10 minutes
Cooking time: 0 minutes
Servings: 5

Ingredients:
- 1 cup heavy cream
- A pinch of salt
- 1 teaspoon stevia
- ½ cup lemon juice
- 8 ounces mascarpone cheese

Directions:
In a bowl, mix the heavy cream with the mascarpone and lemon juice, and stir using a mixer. Add a pinch of salt, and stevia, and blend everything. Divide into dessert glasses and keep in the refrigerator until ready to serve.

Nutrition: Calories - 265, Fat - 27, Fiber - 0, Carbs - 2, Protein - 4

Vanilla Ice Cream

Preparation time: 3 hours and 10 minutes
Cooking time: 0 minutes
Servings: 6

Ingredients:
- 4 eggs, yolks, and whites separated
- ¼ teaspoon cream of tartar
- ½ cup swerve
- 1 tablespoon vanilla extract
- 1¼ cup heavy whipping cream

Directions:
In a bowl, mix the egg whites with the cream of tartar and swerve and stir using a mixer. In another bowl, whisk the cream with the vanilla extract and blend well. Combine the 2 mixtures and stir gently. In another bowl, whisk the egg yolks well and then add the two egg whites mixture. Stir gently, pour the mixture into a container, and keep in the freezer for 3 hours before serving.

Nutrition: Calories - 243, Fat - 22, Fiber - 0, Carbs - 2, Protein - 4

Cheesecake Squares

Preparation time: 10 minutes
Cooking time: 20 minutes
Servings: 9

Ingredients:
- 5 ounces coconut oil, melted
- ½ teaspoon baking powder
- 4 tablespoons swerve
- 1 teaspoon vanilla extract
- 4 ounces cream cheese
- 6 eggs
- ½ cup blueberries

Directions:
In a bowl, mix the coconut oil with the eggs, cream cheese, vanilla extract, swerve, and baking powder and blend using an immersion blender. Fold the blueberries, pour everything into a square baking dish, place in an oven at 320°F, and bake for 20 minutes. Let the cake cool down, slice into squares, and serve.

Nutrition: Calories - 220, Fat - 2, Fiber - 0. 5, Carbs - 2, Protein - 4

Brownies

Preparation time: 10 minutes
Cooking time: 20 minutes
Servings: 12

Ingredients:
- 6 ounces coconut oil, melted
- 6 eggs
- 3 ounces cocoa powder
- 2 teaspoons vanilla extract
- ½ teaspoon baking powder
- 4 ounces cream cheese
- 5 tablespoons swerve

Directions:
In a blender, mix the eggs with the coconut oil, cocoa powder, baking powder, vanilla extract, cream cheese, and swerve and stir using a mixer. Pour this into a lined baking dish, place in an oven at 350°F, and bake for 20 minutes. Cool for awhile, slice into rectangle pieces, and serve.

Nutrition: Calories - 178, Fat - 14, Fiber - 2, Carbs - 3, Protein - 5

Chocolate Pudding

Preparation time: 50 minutes
Cooking time: 5 minutes
Servings: 2

Ingredients:
- 2 tablespoons water
- 1 tablespoon gelatin
- 2 tablespoons maple syrup
- ½ teaspoon stevia powder
- 2 tablespoons cocoa powder
- 1 cup coconut milk

Directions:
Heat up a pan with the coconut milk over medium heat, add the stevia and cocoa powder, and stir well. In a bowl, mix the gelatin with water, stir well, and add to the pan. Stir well, add the maple syrup, whisk again, divide into ramekins, and keep in the refrigerator for 45 minutes. Serve cold.

Nutrition: Calories - 140, Fat - 2, Fiber - 2, Carbs - 4, Protein - 4

Vanilla Parfaits

Preparation time: 10 minutes
Cooking time: 0 minutes
Servings: 4

Ingredients:
- 14 ounces canned coconut milk
- 1 teaspoon vanilla extract
- 10 drops stevia
- 4 ounces berries
- 2 tablespoons walnuts, chopped

Directions:
In a bowl, mix the coconut milk with stevia and vanilla extract, and whisk using a mixer. In another bowl, mix the berries with walnuts, and stir. Spoon half of the vanilla coconut mixture into 4 jars, add a layer of berries, and top with the rest of the vanilla mixture. Top with berries and walnuts mixture, place in the refrigerator to chill before serving.

Nutrition: Calories - 400, Fat - 23, Fiber - 4, Carbs - 6, Protein - 7

Avocado Pudding

Preparation time: 10 minutes
Cooking time: 0 minutes
Servings: 4

Ingredients:
- 2 avocados, pitted, peeled, and chopped
- 2 teaspoons vanilla extract
- 80 drops stevia
- 1 tablespoon lime juice
- 14 ounces canned coconut milk

Directions:
In a blender, mix the avocado with coconut milk, vanilla extract, stevia, and lime juice, blend well, spoon into dessert bowls, and keep in the refrigerator until ready to serve it.

Nutrition: Calories - 150, Fat - 3, Fiber - 3, Carbs - 5, Protein - 6

Mint Delight

Preparation time: 2 hours and 10 minutes
Cooking time: 0 minutes
Servings: 3

Ingredients:
- ½ cup coconut oil, melted
- 3 stevia drops
- 1 tablespoon cocoa powder
- 1 teaspoon peppermint oil
- 14 ounces canned coconut milk
- 1 avocado, pitted, peeled, and chopped
- 10 drops stevia

For the pudding:

Directions:
In a bowl, mix the coconut oil with the cocoa powder and 3 drops stevia, stir well, transfer to a lined container, and keep in the refrigerator for 1 hour. Chop this into small pieces, and set aside. In a blender, mix the coconut milk with avocado, 10 drops stevia, and peppermint oil, and pulse well. Add the chocolate chips, fold them gently, divide pudding into bowls, and keep in the refrigerator for an hour.

Nutrition: Calories - 140, Fat - 3, Fiber - 2, Carbs - 3, Protein - 4

Coconut Pudding

Preparation time: 10 minutes
Cooking time: 10 minutes
Servings: 4

Ingredients:
- 1, and ⅔ cups coconut milk
- 1 tablespoon gelatin
- 6 tablespoons swerve
- 3 egg yolks
- ½ teaspoon vanilla extract

Directions:
In a bowl, mix the gelatin with 1 tablespoon coconut milk, stir well, and set aside. Put the rest of the milk into a pan and heat up over medium heat. Add the swerve, stir, and cook for 5 minutes. In a bowl, mix the egg yolks with the hot coconut milk, and vanilla extract, stir well, and return everything to the pan. Cook for 4 minutes, add the gelatin, and stir well. Divide this into 4 ramekins, and keep the pudding in the refrigerator until you serve it.

Nutrition: Calories - 140, Fat - 2, Fiber - 0, Carbs - 2, Protein - 2

Creamy Coconut Pudding

Preparation time: 4 hours and 10 minutes
Cooking time: 3 minutes
Servings: 2

Ingredients:
- 4 teaspoons gelatin
- ¼ teaspoon liquid stevia
- 1 cup coconut milk
- A pinch of ground cardamom
- ¼ teaspoon ground ginger
- A pinch of ground nutmeg

Directions:
In a bowl, mix the ¼ cup milk with gelatin, and stir well. Put the rest of the coconut milk in a pot and heat up over medium heat. Add the gelatin mixture, stir, take off the heat, set aside to cool down, and then keep in the refrigerator for 4 hours. Transfer this to a food processor, add the stevia, cardamom, nutmeg, and ginger, and blend for a couple of minutes. Divide into dessert cups and serve cold.

Nutrition: Calories - 150, Fat - 1, Fiber - 0, Carbs - 2, Protein - 6

Chocolate Biscotti

Preparation time: 10 minutes
Cooking time: 12 minutes
Servings: 8

Ingredients:
- 2 tablespoons chia seeds
- 2 cups almonds
- 1 egg
- ¼ cup coconut oil
- ¼ cup coconut, shredded
- 2 tablespoons stevia
- ¼ cup cocoa powder
- A pinch of salt
- 1 teaspoon baking soda

Directions:
In a food processor, mix the chia seeds with the almonds and blend well. Add the coconut, egg, coconut oil, cocoa powder, a pinch of salt, baking soda, and stevia, and blend well. Shape 8 biscotti pieces out of this dough, place on a lined baking sheet, place in an oven at 350°F, and bake for 12 minutes. Serve warm or cold.

Nutrition: Calories - 200, Fat - 2, Fiber - 1, Carbs - 3, Protein - 4

Peanut Butter and Chocolate Brownies

Preparation time: 10 minutes
Cooking time: 30 minutes
Servings: 4

Ingredients:
- 1 egg
- ⅓ cup cocoa powder
- ⅓ cup erythritol
- 7 tablespoons butter
- A pinch of salt
- ½ teaspoon vanilla extract
- ¼ cup almond flour
- ¼ cup walnuts
- ½ teaspoon baking powder
- 1 tablespoon peanut butter

Directions:
Heat up a pan with 6 tablespoons butter and the erythritol over medium heat, stir, and cook for 5 minutes. Transfer this to a bowl, add the salt, vanilla extract, and cocoa powder, and whisk. Add the egg, and stir well. Add the baking powder, walnuts, and almond flour, stir well, and pour into a skillet. In a bowl, mix the 1 tablespoon butter with peanut butter, heat up in a microwave for a few seconds, and stir well. Drizzle this over brownies mixture in the skillet, place in an oven at 350ºF, and bake for 30 minutes. Let the brownies to cool down, cut, and serve.

Nutrition: Calories - 223, Fat - 32, Fiber - 1, Carbs - 3, Protein - 6

Blueberry Scones

Preparation time: 10 minutes
Cooking time: 10 minutes
Servings: 10

Ingredients:
- ½ cup coconut flour
- 1 cup blueberries
- 2 eggs
- ½ cup heavy cream
- ½ cup butter
- ½ cup almond flour
- A pinch of salt
- 5 tablespoons stevia
- 2 teaspoons vanilla extract
- 2 teaspoons baking powder

Directions:
In a bowl, mix the almond flour with the coconut flour, salt, baking powder, and blueberries, and stir well. In another bowl, mix the heavy cream with the butter, vanilla extract, stevia, and eggs, and stir well. Combine the 2 mixtures, and stir until you obtain a dough. Shape 10 triangles from this mixture, place them on a lined baking sheet, place in an oven at 350ºF, and bake for 10 minutes. Serve cold.

Nutrition: Calories - 130, Fat - 2, Fiber - 2, Carbs - 4, Protein - 3

Chocolate Cookies

Preparation time: 10 minutes
Cooking time: 40 minutes
Servings: 12

Ingredients:
- 1 teaspoon vanilla extract
- ½ cup butter
- 1 egg
- 2 tablespoons coconut sugar
- ¼ cup swerve
- A pinch of salt
- 2 cups almond flour
- ½ cup unsweetened chocolate chips

Directions:
Heat up a pan with the butter over medium heat, stir, and cook until it browns. Take off the heat, and set aside for 5 minutes. In a bowl, mix the egg with vanilla extract, coconut sugar, and swerve, and stir. Add the melted butter, flour, salt, and half of the chocolate chips, and stir. Transfer this to a pan, spread the rest of the chocolate chips on top, place in an oven at 350ºF, and bake for 30 minutes. Slice when cool and serve.

Nutrition: Calories - 230, Fat - 12, Fiber - 2, Carbs - 4, Protein - 5

Orange Cake

Preparation time: 10 minutes
Cooking time: 20 minutes
Servings: 12

Ingredients:
- 6 eggs
- 1 orange, cut into quarters
- 1 teaspoon vanilla extract
- 1 teaspoon baking powder
- 9 ounces almond meal
- 4 tablespoons swerve
- A pinch of salt
- 2 tablespoons orange zest
- 2 ounces stevia
- 4 ounces cream cheese
- 4 ounces coconut yogurt

Directions:
In a food processor, pulse the orange well. Add the almond meal, swerve, eggs, baking powder, vanilla extract, and a pinch of salt, and pulse well. Transfer this into 2 springform pans, place in an oven at 350°F, and bake for 20 minutes. In a bowl, mix the cream cheese with the orange zest, coconut yogurt, and stevia, and stir well. Place one cake layer on a plate, add the half of the cream cheese mixture, add the other cake layer, and top with the rest of the cream cheese mixture. Spread it well, slice, and serve.

Nutrition: Calories - 200, Fat - 13, Fiber - 2, Carbs - 5, Protein - 8

Walnut Spread

Preparation time: 10 minutes
Cooking time: 0 minutes
Servings: 6

Ingredients:
- 2 ounces coconut oil
- 4 tablespoons cocoa powder
- 1 teaspoon vanilla extract
- 1 cup walnuts, halved
- 4 tablespoons stevia

Directions:
In a food processor, mix the cocoa powder with oil, vanilla extract, walnuts, and stevia, and blend well. Keep in the refrigerator for a couple of hours and serve.

Nutrition: Calories - 100, Fat - 10, Fiber - 1, Carbs - 3, Protein - 2

Mug Cake

Preparation time: 2 minutes
Cooking time: 3 minutes
Servings: 1

Ingredients:
- 4 tablespoons almond meal
- 2 tablespoon butter
- 1 teaspoon stevia
- 1 tablespoon cocoa powder, unsweetened
- 1 egg
- 1 tablespoon coconut flour
- ¼ teaspoon vanilla extract
- ½ teaspoon baking powder

Directions:
Put the butter in a mug and introduce in the microwave for a couple of seconds. Add the cocoa powder, stevia, egg, baking powder, vanilla extract, and coconut flour, and stir well. Add the almond meal as well, stir again, place in the microwave, and cook for 2 minutes. Serve the mug cake with berries on top.

Nutrition: Calories - 450, Fat - 34, Fiber - 7, Carbs - 10, Protein - 20

Sweet Buns

Preparation time: 10 minutes
Cooking time: 30 minutes
Servings: 8

Ingredients:
- ½ cup coconut flour
- ⅓ cup psyllium husks
- 2 tablespoons swerve
- 1 teaspoon baking powder
- A pinch of salt
- ½ teaspoon ground cinnamon
- ½ teaspoon ground cloves
- 4 eggs
- Chocolate chips, unsweetened
- 1 cup hot water

Directions:
In a bowl, mix the flour with psyllium husks, swerve, baking powder, salt, cinnamon, cloves, and chocolate chips, and stir well. Add the water and egg, stir well until you obtain a dough, shape 8 buns, and arrange them on a lined baking sheet. Place in an oven at 350ºF, and bake for 30 minutes, let cool briefly, and serve.

Nutrition: Calories - 100, Fat - 3, Fiber - 3, Carbs - 6, Protein - 6

Lemon Custard

Preparation time: 10 minutes
Cooking time: 30 minutes
Servings: 6

Ingredients:
- 1⅓ pint almond milk
- 4 tablespoons lemon zest
- 4 eggs
- 5 tablespoons swerve
- 2 tablespoons lemon juice

Directions:
In a bowl, mix the eggs with the milk and swerve, and stir well. Add the lemon zest and lemon juice, whisk, pour into ramekins, and place them into a baking dish with some water on the bottom. Bake in the oven at 360ºF for 30 minutes. Let the custard to cool down before serving.

Nutrition: Calories - 120, Fat - 6, Fiber - 2, Carbs - 5, Protein - 7

Chocolate Ganache

Preparation time: 1 minute
Cooking time: 5 minutes
Servings: 6

Ingredients:
- ½ cup heavy cream
- 4 ounces dark chocolate, unsweetened, and chopped

Directions:
Put the cream into a pan and heat up over medium heat. Take off the heat when it begins to simmer, add the chocolate pieces, and stir until it melts. Serve cold as a dessert or use it as a topping for a keto cake.

Nutrition: Calories - 78, Fat - 1, Fiber - 1, Carbs - 2, Protein - 0

Mixed Berries and Cream

Preparation time: 10 minutes
Cooking time: 0 minutes
Servings: 4

Ingredients:
- 3 tablespoons cocoa powder
- 14 ounces heavy cream
- 1 cup blackberries
- 1 cup raspberries
- 2 tablespoons stevia
- Coconut chips

Directions:
In a bowl, whisk the cocoa powder with the stevia and heavy cream. Divide some of this mixture into dessert bowls, add the blackberries, raspberries, and coconut chips, then spread another layer of cream, and top with berries, and chips. Serve cold.

Nutrition: Calories - 245, Fat - 34, Fiber - 2, Carbs - 6, Protein - 2

Coconut Ice Cream

Preparation time: 10 minutes
Cooking time: 0 minutes
Servings: 4

Ingredients:
- 1 mango, sliced
- 14 ounces coconut cream, frozen

Directions:
In a food processor, mix the mango with the cream and pulse well. Divide into bowls and serve.

Nutrition: Calories - 150, Fat - 12, Fiber - 2, Carbs - 6, Protein - 1

Macaroons

Preparation time: 10 minutes
Cooking time: 10 minutes
Servings: 20

Ingredients:
- 2 tablespoons stevia
- 4 egg whites
- 2 cup coconut, shredded
- 1 teaspoon vanilla extract

Directions:
In a bowl, mix the egg whites with stevia and beat using a mixer. Add the coconut and vanilla extract and stir. Roll this mixture into small balls and place them on a lined baking sheet. Place in an oven at 350°F and bake for 10 minutes. Cool and serve.

Nutrition: Calories - 55, Fat - 6, Fiber - 1, Carbs - 2, Protein - 1

Lime Cheesecake

Preparation time: 10 minutes
Cooking time: 2 minutes
Servings: 10

Ingredients:
- 2 tablespoons butter, melted
- 2 teaspoons granulated stevia
- 4 ounces almond meal
- ¼ cup coconut, unsweetened, and shredded
- 1 pound cream cheese
- Zest from 1 lime
- Juice from 1 lime
- 2 sachets sugar-free lime jelly
- 2 cup hot water

For the filling:

Directions:
Heat up a small pan over medium heat, add the butter, and stir until it melts. In a bowl, mix the coconut with the almond meal, butter, and stevia, and stir well. Press this on the bottom of a round pan, and place it in the refrigerator. Put hot water in a bowl, add the jelly sachets, and stir until it dissolves. Put the cream cheese in a bowl, add the jelly, and stir well. Add the lime juice, and lime zest and blend using a mixer. Pour this over the base, spread, and keep the cheesecake in the refrigerator until you serve it.

Nutrition: Calories - 300, Fat - 23, Fiber - 2, Carbs - 5, Protein - 7

Coconut and Strawberries

Preparation time: 10 minutes
Cooking time: 0 minutes
Servings: 4

Ingredients:
- 1¾ cups coconut cream
- 2 teaspoons granulated stevia
- 1 cup strawberries

Directions:
Put the coconut cream in a bowl, add the stevia, and stir well using an immersion blender. Add the strawberries, fold them gently into the mixture, divide dessert into glasses, and serve them cold.

Nutrition: Calories - 245, Fat - 24, Fiber - 1, Carbs - 5, Protein - 4

Caramel Custard

Preparation time: 10 minutes
Cooking time: 30 minutes
Servings: 2

Ingredients:
- 1½ teaspoons caramel extract
- 1 cup water
- 2 ounces cream cheese
- 2 eggs
- 1½ tablespoons swerve

For the caramel sauce:
- 2 tablespoons swerve
- 2 tablespoons butter
- ¼ teaspoon caramel extract

Directions:
In a blender, mix the cream cheese with the water, 1½ tablespoons swerve, 1½ teaspoons caramel extract, and eggs, and blend well. Pour this into 2 greased ramekins, place in an oven at 350°F and bake for 30 minutes. Put the butter in a pot and heat up over medium heat. Add ¼ teaspoon caramel extract and 2 tablespoons swerve, stir well, and cook until everything melts. Pour this over caramel custard, let cool, and serve.

Nutrition: Calories - 254, Fat - 24, Fiber - 1, Carbs - 2, Protein - 8

Cookie Dough Balls

Preparation time: 10 minutes
Cooking time: 0 minutes
Servings: 10

Ingredients:
- ½ cup almond butter
- 3 tablespoons coconut flour
- 3 tablespoons coconut milk
- 1 teaspoon ground cinnamon, powder
- 3 tablespoons coconut sugar
- 15 drops stevia
- A pinch of salt
- 1 teaspoon vanilla extract

For the topping:
- 1½ teaspoon ground cinnamon
- 3 tablespoons granulated swerve

Directions:
In a bowl, mix the almond butter with 1 teaspoon ground cinnamon, coconut flour, coconut milk, coconut sugar, vanilla extract, stevia, and a pinch of salt, and stir well. Shape balls out of this mixture. In another bowl, mix 1½ teaspoon cinnamon with the swerve, and stir well. Roll the balls in cinnamon mixture and keep them in the refrigerator until you serve.

Nutrition: Calories - 89, Fat - 1, Fiber - 2, Carbs - 4, Protein - 2

Ricotta Mousse

Preparation time: 2 hours and 10 minutes
Cooking time: 0 minutes
Servings: 10

Ingredients:
- ½ cup hot coffee
- 2 cups ricotta cheese
- 2, and ½ teaspoons gelatin
- 1½ teaspoon vanilla extract
- 1 teaspoon espresso powder
- 1 teaspoon stevia
- A pinch of salt
- 1 cup whipping cream

Directions:
In a bowl, mix the coffee with the gelatin, stir well, and set aside until coffee is cold. In a bowl, mix the espresso, stevia, salt, vanilla extract, and ricotta, and stir using a mixer. Add the coffee mixture, and stir well. Add the whipping cream and blend mixture again. Divide into dessert bowls and serve after chilling in the refrigerator for 2 hours.

Nutrition: Calories - 160, Fat - 13, Fiber - 0, Carbs - 2, Protein - 7

Coconut Granola

Preparation time: 10 minutes
Cooking time: 35 minutes
Servings: 4

Ingredients:
- 1 cup coconut, unsweetened, and shredded
- 1 cup almonds, and pecans, chopped
- 2 tablespoons stevia
- ½ cup pumpkin seeds
- ½ cup sunflower seeds
- 2 tablespoons coconut oil
- 1 teaspoon ground nutmeg
- 1 teaspoon apple pie spice mix

Directions:
In a bowl, mix the almonds, pecans, pumpkin seeds, sunflower seeds, coconut, nutmeg, and apple pie spice mix, and stir well. Heat up a pan with the coconut oil over medium heat, add the stevia, and stir until combined. Pour this over the nuts and coconut mixture and stir well. Spread this on a lined baking sheet, place in an oven at 300°F, and bake for 30 minutes. Let the granola cool, then cut and serve.

Nutrition: Calories - 120, Fat - 2, Fiber - 2, Carbs - 4, Protein - 7

Peanut Butter and Chia Pudding

Preparation time: 10 minutes
Cooking time: 0 minutes
Servings: 4

Ingredients:
- ½ cup chia seeds
- 2 cups almond milk, unsweetened
- 1½ teaspoon vanilla extract
- ¼ cup peanut butter, unsweetened
- 1 teaspoon stevia
- A pinch of salt

Directions:
In a bowl, mix the milk with the chia seeds, peanut butter, vanilla extract, stevia, and pinch of salt, and stir well. Let the this pudding aside for 5 minutes, stir it again, divide into dessert glasses, and leave in the refrigerator for 10 minutes before serving.

Nutrition: Calories - 120, Fat - 1, Fiber - 2, Carbs - 4, Protein - 2

Pumpkin Custard

Preparation time: 10 minutes
Cooking time: 5 minutes
Servings: 6

Ingredients:
- 1 tablespoon gelatin
- ¼ cup warm water
- 14 ounces canned coconut milk
- 14 ounces canned pumpkin puree
- A pinch of salt
- 2 teaspoons vanilla extract
- 1 teaspoon ground cinnamon
- 1 teaspoon pumpkin pie spice
- 8 scoops stevia
- 3 tablespoons erythritol

Directions:
In a pot, mix the pumpkin puree with the coconut milk, a pinch of salt, vanilla extract, cinnamon, stevia, erythritol, and pumpkin pie spice, stir well, and heat up for a couple of minutes. In a bowl, mix the gelatin, and water, and stir. Combine the 2 mixtures, stir well, divide the custard into ramekins, and set aside to cool down. Keep in the refrigerator until ready to serve.

Nutrition: Calories - 200, Fat - 2, Fiber - 1, Carbs - 3, Protein - 5

No-bake Cookies

Preparation time: 40 minutes
Cooking time: 2 minutes
Servings: 4

Ingredients:
- 1 cup swerve
- ¼ cup coconut milk
- ¼ cup coconut oil
- 2 tablespoons cocoa powder
- 1¾ cup coconut, shredded
- ½ teaspoon vanilla extract
- A pinch of salt
- ¾ cup almond butter

Directions:
Heat up a pan with the oil over medium-high heat, add the milk, cocoa powder, and swerve, stir well for about 2 minutes, and take off the heat. Add the vanilla extract, a pinch of salt, coconut, and almond butter, and stir well. Place spoonful of this mixture on a lined baking sheet, keep in the refrigerator for 30 minutes, and then serve them.

Nutrition: Calories - 150, Fat - 2, Fiber - 1, Carbs - 3, Protein - 6

Butter Delight

Preparation time: 10 minutes
Cooking time: 4 minutes
Servings: 16

Ingredients:
- 4 ounces coconut butter
- 4 ounces cocoa butter
- ¼ cup swerve
- ½ cup peanut butter
- 4 ounces dark chocolate, sugar free
- ½ teaspoon vanilla extract
- ⅛ teaspoon xanthan gum

Directions:
Put the coconut butter, cocoa butter, peanut butter, and swerve in a pan, and heat up over medium heat. Stir until combined, and then mix with the xanthan gum and vanilla extract. Stir well, pour into a lined baking sheet, and spread in a pan. Keep this in the refrigerator for 10 minutes. Heat up a pot with water over medium-high heat and bring to a simmer. Add a bowl on top of the pan, and add chocolate to the bowl. Stir until it melts and drizzle this over the butter mixture. Keep in the refrigerator until everything is firm, cut into 16 pieces, and serve.

Nutrition: Calories - 176, Fat - 15, Fiber - 2, Carbs - 5, Protein - 3

Marshmallows

Preparation time: 10 minutes
Cooking time: 3 minutes
Servings: 6

Ingredients:
- 2 tablespoons gelatin
- 12 scoops stevia
- ½ cup cold water
- ½ cup hot water
- 2 teaspoons vanilla extract
- ¾ cup erythritol

Directions:
In a bowl, mix the gelatin with the cold water, stir, and set aside for 5 minutes. Put the hot water in a pan, add the erythritol and stevia, and stir well. Combine this with the gelatin mixture, add the vanilla extract, and stir well. Beat using a mixer and pour into a baking pan. Set aside in the refrigerator until it sets, then cut into pieces, and serve.

Nutrition: Calories - 140, Fat - 2, Fiber - 1, Carbs - 2, Protein - 4

Tiramisu Pudding

Preparation time: 2 hours and 10 minutes
Cooking time: 0 minutes
Servings: 1

Ingredients:
- 8 ounces cream cheese
- 16 ounces cottage cheese
- 2 tablespoons cocoa powder
- 1 teaspoon instant coffee
- 4 tablespoons almond milk
- 1½ cup sucralose

Directions:
In a food processor, mix the cottage cheese with the cream cheese, cocoa powder, and coffee, and blend well. Add the sucralose and almond milk, blend again, and divide into dessert cups. Keep in the refrigerator until you are ready to serve.

Nutrition: Calories - 200, Fat - 2, Fiber - 2, Carbs - 5, Protein - 5

Summer Smoothie

Preparation time: 5 minutes
Cooking time: 0 minutes
Servings: 2

Ingredients:
- ½ cup coconut milk
- 1½ cup avocado, pitted and peeled
- 2 tablespoons green tea powder
- 2 teaspoons lime zest
- 1 tablespoon coconut sugar
- 1 mango sliced thin, for serving

Directions:
In a smoothie maker, combine the milk with the avocado, green tea powder, and lime zest, and pulse well. Add the sugar, blend well, divide into 2 glasses, and serve with mango slices on top.

Nutrition: Calories - 87, Fat - 5, Fiber - 3, Carbs - 6, Protein - 8

Lemon Sorbet

Preparation time: 5 minutes
Cooking time: 0 minutes
Servings: 4

Ingredients:
- 4 cups ice
- Stevia, to taste
- 1 lemon, peeled, and chopped

Directions:
In a blender, mix the lemon piece with the stevia and ice, and blend until everything is combined. Divide into glasses and serve cold.

Nutrition: Calories - 67, Fat - 0, Fiber - 0, Carbs - 1, Protein - 1

Raspberry Ice Pops

Preparation time: 2 hours
Cooking time: 10 minutes
Servings: 4

Ingredients:
- 1½ cups raspberries
- 2 cups water

Directions:
Put the raspberries, and water in a pan, bring to a boil, and simmer for 10 minutes at medium heat. Pour the mixture into an ice cube tray, stick ice pop sticks into each one, and freeze for 2 hours.

Nutrition: Calories - 60, Fat - 0, Fiber - 0, Carbs - 0, Protein - 2

Cherry and Chia Jam

Preparation time: 15 minutes
Cooking time: 12 minutes
Servings: 22

Ingredients:
- 3 tablespoons chia seeds
- 2, and ½ cups cherries, pitted
- ½ teaspoon vanilla extract
- Peel from ½ lemon, grated
- ¼ cup erythritol
- 10 drops stevia
- 1 cup water

Directions:
Put the cherries and water in a pot, add the stevia, erythritol, vanilla extract, chia seeds, and lemon peel, stir, bring to a simmer, and cook for 12 minutes. Take off the heat and set the jam aside for 15 minutes at least. Serve cold.

Nutrition: Calories - 60, Fat - 1, Fiber - 1, Carbs - 2, Protein - 0. 5

Conclusion

This is really a life-changing cookbook. It shows you everything you need to know about the ketogenic diet, and it helps you get started.

You now know some of the best and most popular ketogenic recipes in the world. We have something here for everyone's taste.

So, don't hesitate too much, and start your new life as a follower of the ketogenic diet. Get your hands on this special recipes collection, and start cooking in this new, exciting and healthy way.

Have a lot of fun and enjoy your ketogenic diet lifestyle!

Recipe Index

A
Almond Butter Bars, 84
Almond Cereal, 23
Almond Pancakes, 30
Apple Salad, 49
Artichoke Dip, 93
Arugula and Broccoli Soup, 176
Arugula Salad, 175
Arugula Soup, 175
Asian Salad, 50
Asian Side Salad, 72
Asparagus and Browned Butter, 170
Asparagus Fries, 170
Asparagus Frittata, 170
Avocado and Bacon Soup, 174
Avocado and Cucumber Salad, 174
Avocado and Egg Salad, 173
Avocado Dip, 82
Avocado Fries, 58
Avocado Muffins, 26
Avocado Pudding, 188
Avocado Salad, 173
Avocado Salsa, 92
Avocado Soup, 174

B
Baby Mushrooms, 74
Bacon and Lemon Thyme Muffins, 26
Bacon and Mushrooms Skewers, 51
Bacon and Zucchini Noodles Salad, 39
Bacon Delight, 89
Bacon-wrapped Chicken, 131
Bacon-wrapped Sausages, 52
Baked Calamari and Shrimp, 104
Baked Chia Seeds, 81
Baked Eggplant Side Salad, 65
Baked Eggs with Sausage, 21
Baked Granola, 31
Baked Haddock, 94
Baked Halibut, 97
Baked Halibut with Vegetables, 100
Baked Sausage and Kale, 162
Baked Turkey Delight, 123
Baked Veal and Cabbage, 157
Balsamic Chicken, 137
Beef and Eggplant Casserole, 151
Beef and Sauerkraut Soup, 149
Beef and Tomato-stuffed Squash, 146
Beef Bourguignon, 157
Beef Brisket Burgers, 38
Beef Chili, 147
Beef Goulash, 151
Beef Jerky, 85
Beef Meatball Casserole, 146
Beef Patties, 145
Beef Pot Roast, 145
Beef Shank Stew, 53
Beef Stew, 158
Beef with Tzatziki, 148
Beef Zucchini Cups, 145
Berry Mousse, 185
Blueberry Scones, 190
Bok Choy Soup, 165
Bok Choy Stir-fry, 165
Braised Asian Eggplant, 75
Braised Lamb Chops, 152
Breadless Breakfast Sandwich, 25
Breadsticks, 87
Breakfast Bowl, 16
Breakfast Bread, 24
Breakfast Casserole, 20
Breakfast Hash, 27
Breakfast in a Glass, 32
Breakfast Meatloaf, 34
Breakfast Muffins, 24
Breakfast Pie, 19
Breakfast Salad in a Jar, 35
Breakfast Skillet, 20
Breakfast Stir-fry, 20
Breakfast Tuna Salad, 35
Broccoli and Cheddar Biscuits, 83
Broccoli Soup, 47
Broccoli Stew, 164
Broccoli Sticks, 88
Broccoli with Lemon Almond Butter, 61
Broiled Brussels Sprouts, 57
Brownies, 187
Brussels Sprout Delight, 28
Brussels Sprout Gratin, 49
Brussels Sprouts and Bacon, 58
Burgundy Beef Stew, 159
Burrito, 27
Butter Delight, 197

C
Cabbage Soup, 181
Calamari Salad, 107
Caprese Salad, 54
Caramel Custard, 194
Caramelized Bell Peppers, 67
Caramelized Red Chard, 67
Catalan-style Greens, 178
Cauliflower Mash, 56
Cauliflower Polenta, 73
Cauliflower Side Salad, 76
Caviar Salad, 91
Celery Soup, 166

Celery Stew, 166
Celery Sticks, 85
Cereal Nibs, 28
Cheddar Soufflés, 75
Cheese and Oregano Muffins, 26
Cheese and Pesto Terrine, 92
Cheese Dough Pizza, 37
Cheese Fries, 90
Cheese Sauce, 70
Cheese Sticks, 88
Cheeseburger Muffins, 79
Cheesecake Squares, 187
Cheesy Chicken, 129
Cherry and Chia Jam, 198
Chia Pudding, 28
Chicken and Broccoli Casserole, 127
Chicken and Shrimp, 53
Chicken and Vegetable Stew, 139
Chicken Breakfast Muffins, 25
Chicken Calzone, 134
Chicken Casserole, 126
Chicken Chowder, 44
Chicken Crepes, 128
Chicken Egg Rolls, 89
Chicken Fajitas, 120
Chicken Gumbo, 133
Chicken in Creamy Sauce, 131
Chicken Meatballs, 118
Chicken Meatloaf, 136
Chicken Nuggets, 117
Chicken Omelet, 33
Chicken Pasta, 138
Chicken Pie, 130
Chicken Quiche, 33
Chicken Salad, 40
Chicken Stew, 139
Chicken Stroganoff, 132
Chicken Thighs with Mushrooms and Cheese, 133
Chicken Wings with Mint Chutney, 117
Chicken with Green Onion Sauce, 136
Chicken with Mustard Sauce, 125
Chicken with Olive Tapenade, 121
Chicken with Sour Cream Sauce, 132
Chicken-stuffed Avocados, 137
Chicken-stuffed Mushrooms, 137
Chicken-stuffed Peppers, 126
Chili Lime Chips, 93
Chili Pepper Burger, 39
Chimichurri Steak Salad, 41
Chocolate Biscotti, 189
Chocolate Bombs, 182
Chocolate Cookies, 190
Chocolate Cups, 185
Chocolate Ganache, 192

Chocolate Pie, 184
Chocolate Pudding, 187
Chocolate Truffles, 182
Chorizo and Cauliflower Breakfast, 22
Clam Chowder, 105
Coconut and Strawberries, 194
Coconut Granola, 195
Coconut Ice Cream, 193
Coconut Pudding, 189
Coconut Shrimp, 101
Coconut Soup, 44
Cod Salad, 108
Cod with Arugula, 99
Coleslaw, 68
Collard Greens and Ham, 167
Collard Greens and Poached Eggs, 168
Collard Greens and Tomatoes, 167
Collard Greens Soup, 168
Collard Greens with Turkey, 60
Cookie Dough Balls, 195
Corndogs, 83
Crab Dip, 86
Cranberry Pork Roast, 142
Cream of Celery Soup, 165
Creamy Asparagus, 171
Creamy Cauliflower and Spinach, 71
Creamy Chicken, 126
Creamy Chicken Soup, 127
Creamy Coconut Pudding, 189
Creamy Radishes, 172
Creamy Spaghetti Pasta, 69
Creamy Spinach, 58
Crispy Radishes, 172
Crusted Chicken, 129
Crusted Salmon, 97
Cuban Beef Stew, 160
Cucumber and Date Salad, 64
Cucumber Cups, 90

D

Doughnuts, 182
Duck Breast Salad, 122
Duck Breast with Vegetables, 121

E

Easy Baked Chicken, 118
Easy Crab Cakes, 42
Easy Grilled Onions, 61
Easy Stuffed Avocado, 41
Easy Tamarind Chutney, 66
Egg Chips, 93
Eggplant and Tomatoes, 60
Eggplant Salad, 64
Eggplant Soup, 180
Eggplant Stew, 180
Eggs and Sausages, 16

Eggs Baked in Avocados, 18
Endive and Watercress Side Salad, 65

F
Fennel and Chicken Salad, 40
Feta and Asparagus Delight, 18
Feta Omelet, 34
Fiery Oysters, 106
Fish Curry, 100
Fish Pie, 94
Flaxseed and Almond Muffins, 80
Flounder and Shrimp, 105
Four-cheese Chicken, 128
Fried Asparagus, 49
Fried Cabbage, 68
Fried Calamari with Spicy Sauce, 104
Fried Chicken, 134
Fried Chicken with Paprika Sauce, 119
Fried Queso, 80
Fried Swiss Chard, 62
Frittata, 17

G
Garlic Spinach Dip, 86
Garlicky Mussels, 103
Gelatin, 183
Glazed Beef Meatloaf, 147
Granola, 23
Greek Side Salad, 63
Green Bean Casserole, 48
Green Beans and Avocado, 68
Green Beans Salad, 47
Green Beans with Vinaigrette, 75
Green Crackers, 92
Green Salad, 177
Green Soup, 54
Grilled Chicken Wings, 118
Grilled Salmon, 98
Grilled Shrimp, 107
Grilled Squid with Guacamole, 112
Grilled Swordfish, 116
Ground Beef Casserole, 149

H
Halibut Soup, 55
Halloumi Salad, 52
Ham Stew, 160
Hemp Porridge, 29
Herbed Biscuits, 25

I
Indian Coconut Chutney, 66
Indian Mint Chutney, 66
Indian Side Salad, 65
Irish Clams, 110
Italian Chicken, 119
Italian Chicken, 125

Italian Clams Delight, 108
Italian Meatballs, 87
Italian Pork Chops, 144
Italian Pork Rolls, 141
Italian Sausage Soup, 163
Italian Spaghetti Casserole, 22

J
Jalapeño Balls, 79
Jalapeño Crisps, 90
Jamaican Beef Pies, 150
Jamaican Pork, 142
Juicy Pork Chops, 142

K
Kiwi and Pineapple Smoothie, 32

L
Lamb Casserole, 155
Lamb Curry, 154
Lamb Riblets and Mint Pesto, 156
Lamb Salad, 152
Lamb Stew, 154
Lamb with Fennel and Figs, 157
Lamb with Mustard Sauce, 153
Lamb with Orange Dressing, 156
Lavender Lamb Chops, 155
Lemon and Garlic Pork, 142
Lemon Chicken, 119
Lemon Custard, 192
Lemon Mousse, 186
Lemon Pork Chops, 143
Lemon Sorbet, 198
Lime Cheesecake, 194
Lobster Bisque, 52
Lunch Caesar Salad, 36
Lunch Curry, 45
Lunch Muffins, 42
Lunch Pâte, 43
Lunch Pizza, 36
Lunch Tacos, 36

M
Macaroons, 193
Maple and Pecan Bars, 81
Marinated Eggs, 77
Marinated Kebabs, 91
Marshmallows, 197
Meatball Pilaf, 47
Meatballs with Mushroom Sauce, 148
Mediterranean Pork, 143
Mexican Breakfast, 19
Mexican Casserole, 50
Mexican Chicken Soup, 135
Mini Bell Pepper Nachos, 83
Mini Cheesecakes, 184
Mint Delight, 188

Mixed Berries and Cream, 193
Mixed Vegetable Dish, 73
Moroccan Lamb, 153
Mug Cake, 191
Mushroom and Hemp Pilaf, 72
Mushroom Salad, 62
Mushrooms and Spinach, 59
Mussel Soup, 114
Mustard and Garlic Brussels Sprouts, 70
Mustard Greens and Spinach Soup, 169
Mustard-glazed Salmon, 113

N
Naan Bread and Butter, 35
No-bake Cookies, 196
Nutty Breakfast Bowl, 23
Nutty Breakfast Smoothie, 32

O
Octopus Salad, 104
Okra and Tomatoes, 59
One-pot Roasted Chicken, 136
Onion and Cauliflower Dip, 77
Orange Cake, 191
Orange Chicken, 130
Orange-glazed Salmon, 109
Oven-fried Green Beans, 56
Oysters with Pico De Gallo, 111

P
Pancakes, 30
Pan-roasted Cod, 99
Pan-seared Duck Breast, 121
Paprika Lamb Chops, 156
Parmesan Wings, 88
Peanut Butter and Chia Pudding, 196
Peanut Butter and Chocolate Brownies, 190
Peanut Butter Fudge, 186
Peanut-grilled Chicken, 138
Pecan-crusted Chicken, 133
Pepperoni Bombs, 79
Pepperoni Chicken Bake, 134
Pesto, 57
Pesto Chicken Salad, 41
Pesto Crackers, 78
Pizza Dip, 80
Pizza Rolls, 37
Poached Eggs, 16
Pork Chops with Mushrooms, 141
Pork Pie, 43
Pork Stew, 158
Porridge, 22
Portobello Mushrooms, 57
Prosciutto-wrapped Shrimp, 82
Pumpkin Custard, 196
Pumpkin Muffins, 78
Pumpkin Pancakes, 30

Pumpkin Soup, 48
Puréed Broccoli and Cauliflower, 164

R
Radish Hash Browns, 172
Radish Soup, 173
Raspberry and Coconut Dessert, 185
Raspberry Ice Pops, 198
Red-hot Chicken Wings, 131
Rice with Cauliflower, 76
Ricotta Mousse, 195
Roasted Asparagus, 169
Roasted Bell Peppers Soup, 180
Roasted Cauliflower, 59
Roasted Mahi Mahi and Salsa, 102
Roasted Olives, 69
Roasted Pork Belly, 140
Roasted Pork Sausage, 162
Roasted Radishes, 171
Roasted Salmon, 96
Roasted Sea Bass, 101
Roasted Tomato Cream, 179

S
Salmon Bites with Chili Sauce, 110
Salmon Meatballs, 96
Salmon Rolls, 106
Salmon Skewers, 107
Salmon Soup, 54
Salmon Stuffed with Shrimp, 113
Salmon with Arugula and Cabbage, 113
Salmon with Caper Sauce, 96
Salmon with Lemon Relish, 114
Salsa Chicken, 125
Sardine Salad, 108
Saucy Zucchini, 84
Sausage and Cheese Dip, 77
Sausage and Peppers Soup, 163
Sausage Gravy, 72
Sausage Patties, 21
Sausage Quiche, 21
Sausage Salad, 163
Sausage Stew, 159
Sausage Stuffing, 74
Sausage with Tomatoes and Cheese, 162
Sautéed Broccoli, 61
Sautéed Kohlrabi, 70
Sautéed Lemon Shrimp, 100
Sautéed Mustard Greens, 167
Sautéed Mustard Greens, 168
Sautéed Zucchini, 62
Savory Chicken, 132
Scallops with Fennel Sauce, 114
Scrambled Eggs, 17
Sea Bass with Capers, 99
Seared Scallops with Walnuts and Grapes, 111

Seasoned Hard-boiled Eggs, 18
Shrimp Alfredo, 103
Shrimp and Bacon Breakfast, 19
Shrimp and Cauliflower, 112
Shrimp and Noodle Salad, 101
Shrimp and Snow Pea Soup, 103
Shrimp Pasta, 50
Shrimp Salad, 106
Shrimp Stew, 102
Simple Breakfast Cereal, 29
Simple Buffalo Wings, 51
Simple Chicken Stir-fry, 135
Simple Egg Porridge, 29
Simple French Toast, 31
Simple Grilled Oysters, 97
Simple Hummus, 85
Simple Kimchi, 56
Simple Smoothie Bowl, 34
Simple Tomato Soup, 51
Simple Tomato Tarts, 82
Skillet Chicken and Mushrooms, 120
Slow-cooked Leg of Lamb, 155
Slow-roasted Beef, 158
Smoked Salmon Breakfast, 17
Snap Peas and Mint, 60
Sour Cream Salmon, 98
Special Tortilla Chips, 78
Spicy Pork Chops, 144
Spicy Shrimp, 102
Spinach and Artichoke Chicken, 135
Spinach Balls, 86
Spinach Rolls, 46
Spinach Soup, 166
Spring Greens Soup, 169
Steak and Eggs, 33
Steak Bowl, 46
Steak Salad, 40
Strawberry Pie, 183
Stuffed Chicken Breast, 124
Stuffed Mushrooms, 87
Stuffed Peppers, 38
Stuffed Pork, 140
Summer Kale, 67
Summer Side Salad, 63
Summer Smoothie, 198
Sushi Bowl, 115
Sweet Buns, 192
Swiss Chard and Chicken Soup, 178
Swiss Chard and Vegetable Soup, 179
Swiss Chard Pie, 177
Swiss Chard Salad, 177
Swordfish with Mango Salsa, 115

T

Taco Cups, 89
Taco Salad, 38
Thai Avocado Soup, 175
Thai Beef, 144
Tilapia, 95
Tiramisu Pudding, 197
Tomato and Bocconcini, 64
Tomato Salsa, 63
Trout with Butter Sauce, 95
Trout with Special Sauce, 95
Tuna and Chimichurri Sauce, 109
Tuna Cakes, 98
Turkey and Cranberry Salad, 124
Turkey and Tomato Curry, 124
Turkey Breakfast, 27
Turkey Chili, 123
Turkey Pie, 122
Turkey Soup, 123
Turnip Fries, 71
Twice-baked Zucchini, 71

V

Vanilla Ice Cream, 186
Vanilla Parfaits, 188
Veal Parmesan, 161
Veal Piccata, 161
Veal Stew, 160
Veal with Tomatoes, 161
Vegetable Breakfast Bread, 24
Vegetable Noodles, 69

W

Waffles, 31
Walnut Spread, 191
Watercress Soup, 164

Z

Zucchini and Avocado Soup, 176
Zucchini Chips, 84
Zucchini Cream, 176
Zucchini Noodles and Beef, 150
Zucchini Noodles Soup, 45
Zucchini Rolls, 91
Zucchini with Cheese, 39

Copyright 2017 by Emily Willis All rights reserved.

All rights Reserved. No part of this publication or the information in it may be quoted from or reproduced in any form by means such as printing, scanning, photocopying or otherwise without prior written permission of the copyright holder.

Disclaimer and Terms of Use: Effort has been made to ensure that the information in this book is accurate and complete, however, the author and the publisher do not warrant the accuracy of the information, text and graphics contained within the book due to the rapidly changing nature of science, research, known and unknown facts and internet. The Author and the publisher do not hold any responsibility for errors, omissions or contrary interpretation of the subject matter herein. This book is presented solely for motivational and informational purposes only.

Made in the USA
San Bernardino, CA
04 January 2018